Integrating a Social Determinants of Health Framework into Nursing Education

Jill B. Hamilton • Beth Ann Swan
Linda McCauley

Editors

Integrating a Social Determinants of Health Framework into Nursing Education

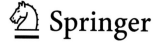 Springer

Editors
Jill B. Hamilton
Nell Hodgson Woodruff School of Nursing
Emory University
Atlanta, GA, USA

Beth Ann Swan
Emory Nursing Learning Center, Nell
Hodgson Woodruff School of Nursing,
Emory University
Atlanta, GA, USA

Linda McCauley
Nell Hodgson Woodruff School of Nursing
Emory University
Atlanta, GA, USA

ISBN 978-3-031-21346-5   ISBN 978-3-031-21347-2   (eBook)
https://doi.org/10.1007/978-3-031-21347-2

This Springer imprint is published by the registered company Springer Nature Switzerland AG
The registered company address is: Gewerbestrasse 11, 6330 Cham, Switzerland

Foreword

The last decade of nursing education and practice has included multiple research, policy, and practice initiatives to fully recognize the immense influence social determinants of health have on the health and illness experience of human populations. The integration of social determinants of health into nursing education is critical to alleviating health disparities and ultimately improving health outcomes. Nurses can be extremely influential to the global initiative to assuage the suffering from health inequities, poverty, and social marginalization that contributes to disparities in illness and health conditions.

However, major changes in nursing curricula can be challenging for a number of reasons. First, the knowledge of the immensity of social determinants of health is actively growing necessitating the integration of new knowledge on a regular basis. Second, we have an aging nursing faculty workforce who were not taught this content in their nursing programs and therefore need knowledge development in this area to be effective in the classroom and clinical settings. Finally, nursing curricula are packed with new and emerging knowledge on the delivery of care to patients. A common lament from faculty is that there is no room for additional content and/or courses. Faculty are faced with the challenge of teaching or expanding on content on social determinants of health when they feel there is no time to do so.

The authors of this text have written this content to assist readers in understanding the journey that we are taking to seriously address the need for full integration of SDOH into nursing education programs. We hope that it will be an important tool for nursing educators in the quest to prepare a nursing workforce that is equipped to address social determinants of health. The journeys that schools will take will be different, and we welcome feedback from our readers on how helpful this information is for your individual journey. We feel that the Emory School of Nursing 4-pillar SDOH framework is a critical part of the map to teaching strategies in nursing to protect and promote optimal health of the individuals, communities, and societies that we serve.

American Nurses Association   Ernest J. Grant
Silver Spring, MD, USA

Acknowledgments

This book is based on the work and determination of the faculty of the Nell Hodgson Woodruff School of Nursing at Emory University to integrate social determinants of health throughout its prelicensure and advanced practice nursing curricula. We are grateful for the faculty and students who either contributed to the work presented in this text or informed the content necessary for the implementation of SDOH into our courses.

Finally, we would like to acknowledge with gratitude the support from Nell Hodgson Woodruff School of Nursing administrative staff Margie Hutson, Kaye-Ann Sadler, and Shanice Smith and to Connor Swan for the original artwork in Chap. 5.

Contents

1 **Social Determinants of Health: Call for Nursing
   Education Reform**   1
   Linda McCauley

2 **Integrating a Social Determinants of Health Framework
   into Nursing Education**   9
   Jill B. Hamilton

3 **Canvas Faculty Development Site** 55
   Adarsh Char

4 **Curriculum Mapping: Integrating Social Determinants
   of Health Within Nursing Education** 119
   Autherine Abiri, Wanjira Kinuthia, and Elizabeth Downes

5 **SDOH in Action: Exemplars of Incorporating SDOH
   Content in Entry-Level and Advanced-Level Nursing Education** 131
   Beth Ann Swan, Lalita Kaligotla, Autherine Abiri, Lindsey Allen,
   Amy Becklenberg, Christina K. Bhatia, Sofia Biller, Susan Brasher,
   Rasheeta Chandler, DeJuan Charles, Erica Davis, Anneke Demmink,
   Harrison Boyd Diamond, Elizabeth Downes, Rebekah Elting,
   Wendy R. Gibbons, Nicholas A. Giordano, Jill B. Hamilton,
   Caroline Kee, Stephanie Lee, Alyssa Meadows, Lori A. Modly,
   Kenneth Mueller, Caitlyn Plattel, Melissa Poole-Dubin,
   Maria-Bernarda Saavedra, Isake Slaughter, Shaquita Starks,
   Susan L. Swanson, Isabella Upchurch, Jessica Wells, Phyllis Wright,
   and Irene Yang

6 **Evaluating Social Determinants of Health Integration
   in Nursing Curricula** 185
   Lisa Muirhead, Susan Brasher, Rasheeta Chandler,
   and Laura P. Kimble

7   Aligning SDOH Pillars to Learning Outcomes and Assessments..... 197
Wanjira Kinuthia, Autherine Abiri, Jill B. Hamilton, and
Adarsh Char

8   Lessons Learned 211
Jill B. Hamilton, Adarsh Char, Linda McCauley, Autherine Abiri,
Laura Kimble, Lalita Kaligotla, Beth Ann Swan, and Kristy Martyn

Social Determinants of Health: Call for Nursing Education Reform

1

Linda McCauley

Learning Objectives

1. Describe the roots of public health nursing practice in nursing history and how this heritage remains a strong influence on the health of individuals and communities today.
2. Explain how Thomas Frieden's 5-tiered Health Impact Pyramid illustrates the potential impact of nursing interventions that target social determinants of health.
3. Give examples of the successful integration of SDOH knowledge in nursing practice, research, and policy.

Introduction

The past two decades have seen increasing attention paid to the roles that social factors play in determining risk of illness. The World Health Organization's (WHO's) Commission on the Social Determinants of Health (2008) has defined SDOH as "the circumstances in which people are born, grow, live, work and age" and "the fundamental drivers of these conditions" (p. 2) [1]. Generally, social determinants of health refer to broad categories of influence that can affect health-related behaviors and outcomes in multiple domains of life. Knowledge is rapidly expanding in this area, exposing the importance of SDOH in shaping health, including the plausible pathways and biological mechanisms that may explain the broad effects of SDOH [2].

The large influence of SDOH illuminates, in part, the failure of many countries to achieve positive health outcomes among all populations, despite rapid advances in medicine and healthcare. McGinnis, Williams-Russo, and Knickman (2002)

L. McCauley (✉)
Nell Hodgson Woodruff School of Nursing, Emory University, Atlanta, GA, USA
e-mail: Linda.mccauley@emory.edu

© The Author(s), under exclusive license to Springer Nature Switzerland AG 2023
J. B. Hamilton et al. (eds.), *Integrating a Social Determinants of Health Framework into Nursing Education*, https://doi.org/10.1007/978-3-031-21347-2_1

estimated that medical care contributes to only 10–15% of preventable mortality in the USA [3]. In contrast, a meta-analysis of the issue by Galea and colleagues (2011) concluded that, in 2000, the number of US deaths attributable to low education, racial segregation, and low social support was comparable with the number of deaths attributable to myocardial infarction, cerebrovascular disease, and lung cancer, respectively [4].

Nursing History and SDOH

Nursing has long recognized the link between the social context of one's life and the ability to be healthy. Nursing, with its roots in public health, demonstrated that services delivered in homes and neighborhoods where people lived and worked were effective in improving the health of persons in those communities. Lillian Wald first used the term "public health nurse," believing that nurses must address social and economic problems, not simply take care of sick people [5]. Philosophically, Wald believed that public health nursing should involve the health of an entire neighborhood, as well as cooperation among stakeholders and communities, to help improve living conditions. In the last decade, public health nurses have remained the largest sector of the public health workforce, and yet their number is strikingly low given the total number of four million nurses in the USA [6]. A 2012 study estimated there are less than 35,000 nurses working in public health departments [7]. While many nurses work outside acute care settings, it is not known to what extent they practice public health nursing or if their roles include interacting with social agencies to improve SDOH in a population framework.

While no one disputes the value of public health nursing, the latter half of the twentieth century saw an emphasis on medical discovery and hospital care. Investment in the country's public health infrastructure was reduced, and fewer city and county public health departments could maintain a robust nursing workforce to interact with patients in their homes, schools, and communities. The majority of new nursing graduates are now employed by hospital systems and have little-to-no time to focus on the social context of patients' lives. Decreasing hospital length-of-stay also has contributed to nursing having less time to interact with patients and families before discharge and few opportunities to follow up in the community. Even nurses working in ambulatory settings are often in specialty clinics where the emphasis is on managing the disease process. Focusing on tertiary care has caused the profession to lose much of its lens on the importance of SDOH in predicting patients' overall health [8, 9].

Nursing Care to Reduce Health Disparities

The ultimate goal of integrating SDOH content into nursing curricula is to improve health outcomes for all through more nuanced and contextualized nursing care. Nursing curricula have historically concentrated on individual-level factors to improve health and lifestyle behaviors. The prominence of these curricular threads is not surprising given nursing's emphasis on wellness and health promotion. Nurses can play critical roles in supporting patients through behavior change, but it should not stop there. Nurses also need to intervene to reduce barriers to health such as institutional racism in healthcare, inadequate access to food, un- or under-employment, unsafe housing, and social isolation. Nurses must be able to offer health education messaging that is culturally appropriate and tailored as well. While the links between socioeconomic status and health are rarely debated, nurses have limited curricular opportunities to explore how socioeconomic factors such as income, wealth, and education impact a wide range of health issues. Coursework on poverty, healthcare finance, and education are not among the traditional prerequisite coursework for nursing; neither is formal instruction on historical and sociopolitical issues, including racism and segregation. As a result, many nurses have limited awareness of how factors such as racial discrimination, violence, poverty, and trauma can intersect, compound, and influence health over a lifetime.

A cross-cutting challenge in care delivery is developing health system interventions that address the huge influence of racial discrimination and structural racism on people's access to and quality of care [10]. Thomas Frieden's 5-tiered Health Impact Pyramid illustrates this complexity well and demonstrates that the greatest health impacts likely will come from interventions that address socioeconomic factors driving health disparities across multiple conditions [11]. Frieden's pyramid suggests that SDOH interventions stand to have the greatest potential public health benefit, but they need government and civil support to be successful. While these interventions are often political in nature, nursing is well positioned to support public interventions to improve the health profile of populations. Just as nursing students are encouraged to advocate for social change that will advance the profession, they also should feel qualified and confident in advocating for change to benefit health for all. Areas of advocacy might include living wages, reproductive health services, elder care, violence prevention, affordable, and accessible housing, to name a few.

To effectively prepare nurses to advocate for such change, faculty must feel comfortable bringing health policy and politics into the classroom. These conversations can be difficult for nursing faculty who may personally oppose public health-backed policies such as increasing the minimum wage or limiting access to firearms in certain populations. Faculty can navigate this by taking a position of empowered vulnerability, admitting their own ambivalence, while still relaying scientific knowledge and creating a forum for inclusive class discussions. Our nation is at a critical juncture in terms of the politicization of trusted scientific knowledge; nursing faculty must promote a culture of trust for science as a foundation for health education, interventions, and policy, even if they do not agree with its ultimate applications. Furthermore, nursing advocacy requires nursing leaders who are both educated about the issues and politically savvy. Curricula therefore ought to incorporate interdisciplinary content, such as at the intersections of political science or public administration and public health [12].

In addition to curricular reform, nursing educators need scientific evidence that interventions introduced in courses can reduce health disparities in practice. Nursing practice is grounded in evidence, and evidence is in fact emerging for interventions designed to improve population health [10]. However, there is a vast gap between what is traditionally taught and new and emerging findings on how to incorporate SDOH into practice. The structure of nursing education needs to change to include not only the knowledge base on SDOH science but also emerging best practices and evaluation strategies for its translation and dissemination.

More than a decade ago, the National Institutes of Health held a summit [13] organized around the central themes of Science, Practice, and Policy. The NIH explored applications of new knowledge about the determinants of health disparities, disease progression, and outcomes in different populations. As the goal of scientific knowledge is practice improvement, the summit explored the skills that would be necessary to address SDOH in healthcare delivery. It stressed that to ensure the best care for patients and populations, a combination of in-depth background, contextual, and clinical knowledge will be necessary. The summit's Policy topic area referred to the course of action or system of interventions that may be adopted by entities regarding science or practice issues. The NIH underscored that research and science should drive policy discussions, thereby influencing change in how care is delivered, or what is prioritized, within a system.

Nurses stand to play a critical role in promoting SDOH knowledge with the goal of reducing health disparities. It is not enough for nursing educators to understand the science on why the social environment is a powerful determinant of health; they also must know about interventions that have proven effective in reducing disparities and improving human health [10]. Research is being conducted to determine the extent to which the rapid increase in SDOH has influenced clinician behavior. Intervention projects are demonstrating that by changing the way care is delivered, outcomes can be improved [14], primarily on the development of screening and assessment tools to more accurately identify patients' SDOH [10, 15–18].

A recent National Academy of Medicine (2021) report outlined evidence of the importance of primary care and connecting with populations where they live, work, worship, and play [19]. Likewise, evidence in support of community-based partnerships is emerging, but needs to be of higher priority so that we can more effectively change care delivery. The National Institutes of Health (NIH) need to place a higher priority in funding research on SDOH and new models of care delivery. In 2022, the National Institute for Nursing Research (NINR) developed its draft strategic plan for the next 5 years. Two of its three major initiatives deal with the promotion of health equity and reducing structural racism. The NINR will support research on developing and implementing interventions to address SDOH. Specifically, NINR will focus on population-level factors such as environments, behaviors, epigenetics, and social genomics that impact health outcomes. Interventions that address SDOH will be prioritized along with identifying barriers and facilitators to decision-making among different populations. The Institute will encourage research focused on developing, rigorously studying, and implementing multilevel interventions that target the individual, family, social supports, community, population, and policy across the lifespan. This strategic plan is ambitious, but aligns well with larger NIH research initiatives to address the SDOH factors that have been driving health inequities [20].

Call to Action

Knowledge of socioeconomic and related social factors in shaping health has become so compelling that it cannot be ignored insofar as public health and healthcare personnel are concerned [2]. Nursing educators need to face the challenge of preparing clinicians to address the broad array of SDOH and develop strategies that reach beyond services to individual patients. Nurses, as members of the largest sector of the healthcare workforce and the most trusted profession, can play an important role in designing interventions to address the influence of SDOH. With more than four million nurses currently employed in the USA [6], the potential impact of their practice transcends hospital and clinic settings, communities, research, and health policy circles. However, few schools of nursing have fully integrated SDOH into all levels of nursing education [21].

Many nursing professional groups have identified the need to enhance educational threads related to SDOH within all types of nursing education. The 2021 Future of Nursing (FON) report notes the repeated calls for competency-based education on the integration of SDOH into nursing practice, recognizing that SDOH concepts are not currently well integrated into nursing programs [9]. There is a critical need to assess to what degree nurses are educated in these areas. The FON report committee could not find any systematic analysis of the current integration of SDOH concepts into nursing curricula or educational experiences. They noted that most programs include SDOH content in a community or public health courses, but it is typically not integrated thoroughly across the curriculum. They also noted the need for curricular designs that address SDOH content beyond community health rotations [9].

The American Association of Colleges of Nursing (AACN) emphasized the need for standardized SDOH competencies in the 2021 *Essentials* as well [22]. The AACN described the importance of SDOH as a unifying concept across all levels of nursing practice and education, stating:

> The social determinants of health contribute to wide health disparities and inequities in areas such as economic stability, education quality and access, healthcare quality and access, neighborhood and built environment, and social and community context [23]. Nursing practices such as assessment, health promotion, access to care, and patient teaching support improvements in health outcomes. The social determinants of health are closely interrelated with the concepts of diversity, equity, and inclusion, health policy, and communication.

The integration of SDOH as an essential curricular component of both undergraduate and graduate programs is the first step to recognizing how critical this content is to competent nursing practice. Its incorporation should be reflected in accreditation standards and in revisions of curricula throughout nursing programs nationally.

SDOH content should not be limited to a small number of courses, but rather used as consistent threads across curricula. This should involve a top-turn curriculum redesign that builds on the following principles:

- A uniform definition of SDOH.
- A curriculum structure that supports the incorporation of SDOH content.
- Faculty development to assure that a wide breadth of nursing faculty can address concepts and exemplars of SDOH, regardless of their practice settings or clinical specialties.
- Nursing and academic cultures that empower faculty, and build their comfort, in advocating for social and political change.
- Assurance that every course in the curriculum addresses exemplars of SDOH in some manner and that the curriculum committee commits to assuring the curriculum design is indeed implemented.
- Assurance that SDOH concepts are integrated into clinical rotations; that students are given opportunities to explore the contribution of SDOH to the health risks they encounter in practice; and that they can identify how to practice settings should integrate SDOH into standards of care.
- Opportunities and encouragement for students to advocate for policy change that will address systemic issues.

Finally, as nursing moves to an enhanced emphasis on competency-based education, nursing faculty should identify the knowledge base and clinical competencies that would indicate sufficient ability to address SDOH, regardless of clinical setting.

References

1. World Health Organization (WHO). Closing the gap in a generation: health equity through action on the social determinants of health. Geneva: WHO Commission on Social Determinants of Health; 2008.
2. Braveman P, Gottlieb L. The social determinants of health: it's time to consider the causes of the causes. Public Health Rep. 2014;129(Suppl 2):19–31.
3. McGinnis JM, Williams-Russo P, Knickman JR. The case for more active policy attention to health promotion. Health Aff (Millwood). 2002;21:78–93.
4. Galea S, Tracy M, Hoggatt KJ, Dimaggio C, Karpati A. Estimated deaths attributable to social factors in the United States. Am J Public Health. 2011;101:1456–65.
5. Fee E, Bu L. The origins of public health nursing: the Henry Street Visiting Nurse Service. Am J Public Health. 2010;100:1206–7.
6. American Nurses Association (ANA). About ANA. 2020. Nursingworld.org/ana/about-ana
7. Beck AJ, Boulton ML. The public health nurse workforce in U.S. state and local health departments, 2012. Public Health Rep. 2016;131:145–52.
8. Institute of Medicine (IOM). For the public's health: investing in a healthier future. Washington, DC: Committee on Public Health Strategies to Improve Health; 2012.
9. National Academies of Sciences, Engineering, and Medicine (NASEM). The future of nursing 2020–2030: charting a path to achieve health equity. The National Academies Press; 2021.

10. Thornton RL, Glover CM, Cené CW, Glik DC, Henderson JA, Williams DR. Evaluating strategies for reducing health disparities by addressing the social determinants of health. Health Aff (Millwood). 2016;35:1416–23.
11. Frieden TR. A framework for public health action: the health impact pyramid. Am J Public Health. 2010;100:590–5.
12. Lathrop B. Nursing leadership in addressing the social determinants of health. Policy Polit Nurs Pract. 2013;14:41–7.
13. Dankwa-Mullan I, Rhee KB, Williams K, et al. The science of eliminating health disparities: summary and analysis of the NIH summit recommendations. Am J Public Health. 2010;100(Suppl 1):S12–8.
14. Chhabra M, Sorrentino AE, Cusack M, Dichter ME, Montgomery AE, True G. Screening for housing instability: providers' reflections on addressing a social determinant of health. J Gen Intern Med. 2019;34:1213–9.
15. Higginbotham K, Davis Crutcher T, Karp SM. Screening for social determinants of health at well-child appointments: a quality improvement project. Nurs Clin North Am. 2019;54:141–8.
16. Morgenlander MA, Tyrrell H, Garfunkel LC, Serwint JR, Steiner MJ, Schilling S. Screening for social determinants of health in pediatric resident continuity clinic. Acad Pediatr. 2019;19:868–74.
17. Morone J. An integrative review of social determinants of health assessment and screening tools used in pediatrics. J Pediatr Nurs. 2017;37:22–8.
18. Walter LA, Schoenfeld EM, Smith CH, et al. Emergency department-based interventions affecting social determinants of health in the United States: a scoping review. Acad Emerg Med. 2021;28:666–74.
19. National Academies of Sciences, Engineering, and Medicine. Implementing high-quality primary care: rebuilding the foundation of health care. Washington, DC: The National Academies Press; 2021.
20. National Institute of Nursing Research (NINR). The National Institute of Nursing Research 2022–2026 strategic plan. 2022.
21. Porter K, Jackson G, Clark R, Waller M, Stanfill AG. Applying social determinants of health to nursing education using a concept-based approach. J Nurs Educ. 2020;59:293–6.
22. American Association of Colleges of Nursing (AACN). The essentials. AACN; 2021.
23. U.S Department of Health and Human Services. Healthy people 2030. 2022. https://health.gov/healthypeople/priority-areas/social-determinants-health. Accessed 3 Oct 2022.

Integrating a Social Determinants of Health Framework into Nursing Education

2

Jill B. Hamilton

Learning Objectives

1. Describe frequently cited SDOH frameworks.
2. Describe four pillars of Nell Hodgson Woodruff School of Nursing SDOH framework.
3. Discuss the utility of four pillars of Nell Hodgson Woodruff School of Nursing SDOH framework with integration of SDOH into nursing curriculum.

Introduction

In the initial phases of the integration of SDOH into the curriculum of the Nell Hodgson Woodruff School of Nursing, faculty members of the Dean's Educational Council met to discuss strategies for the integration of SDOH content into courses through the curriculum. The Dean's Educational Council consists of both elected and appointed members of the faculty who meet monthly for the purpose of advisement to Dean Linda McCauley on key topics related to the overall functioning of the school. During these initial meetings with the Dean's Educational Council, it became apparent that faculty were aware of the importance of SDOH to the education of our nursing students but also found the numerous SDOH conceptualizations and frameworks confusing. Moreover, even though faculty were knowledgeable of SDOH concepts, they were unsure of which framework and/or concepts were relevant to the discipline of nursing. Our initial goal, therefore, was to identify the most appropriate SDOH framework to guide faculty with the integration of SDOH throughout the didactic and clinical courses in our nursing curriculum.

J. B. Hamilton (✉)
Nell Hodgson Woodruff School of Nursing, Emory University, Atlanta, GA, USA
e-mail: jbhamil@emory.edu

© The Author(s), under exclusive license to Springer Nature Switzerland AG 2023
J. B. Hamilton et al. (eds.), *Integrating a Social Determinants of Health Framework into Nursing Education*, https://doi.org/10.1007/978-3-031-21347-2_2

As lead faculty of the initiative to integrate SDOH content into our nursing curriculum, initial steps were to examine SDOH conceptualizations and frameworks accessible through websites, literature searches, and published books for their utility. An initial analysis of SDOH conceptualizations and/or frameworks suggested their origination likely evolved from the mission and purpose of leading public health organizations and health care agencies, including WHO, CDC, US Department their affiliated organizations. Through this initial analysis, it became apparent that the World Health Organization (WHO) and Healthy People 2030 conceptualizations of SDOH were among those most widely referenced and/or cited. This SDOH conceptualization included "the conditions in which people are born, grow, work, live, and age, and the wider set of forces and systems shaping the conditions of daily life" [1]. We decided to adopt the WHO conceptualization of SDOH for our framework given its inclusion of environments where individuals work, worship, and age. We were also intrigued by the WHO conceptualization it was endorsed by nursing credentialing organizations (American Association of Colleges of Nursing, National League of Nursing) and consistent with our goal of providing optimal nursing care in diverse settings of health care settings; communities, faith-based institutions, and school-based settings among diverse populations.

Review of SDOH Frameworks

Our analysis of frequently cited SDOH frameworks was not as clearly delineated as the conceptualizations to guide the integration of SDOH throughout the curriculum. Rather, SDOH frameworks appeared to be designed or constructed to address the promotion of health for focused issues or the prevention of illness. The following review is of a few frameworks most frequently referenced or cited and our assessment of their utility in guiding the integration of SDOH into our curriculum. Details of these frameworks are published elsewhere and only briefly summarized here.

The World Health Organization's (WHO) Commission on SDOH, for example, published a conceptual framework to guide their mission to promote the highest level of health among global populations [2]. Perhaps the most notable function of this organization is to monitor and respond to public health emergencies and to promote the health and well-being of populations globally. Moreover, the global public health focus of this organization is apparent in its history of leading the world's efforts to eradicate communicable diseases such as HIV/AIDS, COVID-19, and Ebola as well as noncommunicable diseases such as cancer and heart disease.

The Commission on Social Determinants of Health (CSDH) Framework (Fig. 2.1) has two major components: Structural determinants of health inequities and Intermediary determinants of Health. In addition to Structural and Intermediary Determinants, this framework considers that the care delivered is within a socioeconomic and political context which subsequently influences health equity and well-being in positive and negative ways.

Structural determinants refer specifically to one's social stratification and resulting socioeconomic positioning of individuals within a society situated within a

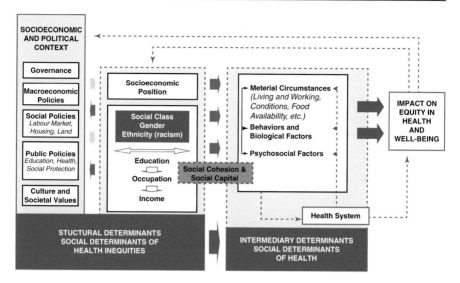

Fig. 2.1 WHO commission on SDOH framework

sociopolitical context (macroeconomic, social, and public policies and cultural and social values). On the other hand, *Intermediary determinants* are defined as those more downstream social determinants such as material circumstances; psychosocial circumstances; behavioral and/or biological factors; and, the health care system. These intermediary differences in health are unequally distributed in society according to one's social class, occupational status, educational achievement, and income level. Intermediary influences may also include aspects of one's physical environment such as housing and the safety of one's home and neighborhood. Psychosocial stressors may be stressful living situations and coping strategies such as social support. Behavioral and/or biological factors may include engaging in unhealthy behaviors such as smoking, lack of physical exercise, alcohol consumption, and genetic factors. The final intermediary determinant in this model is the health care system. As a social determinant of health and intermediary influence, equitable access to the health care system can result in the promotion of health or increased vulnerability to health or illness.

Another major aspect of the CSDH framework is *the socioeconomic-political context* within which the Structural and Intermediary determinants operate. Socioeconomic-political context refers to a range of factors that cannot be directly measured at the individual level and yet exerts a powerful influence on the formation of social classes and individual ability to access health care. For example, a socioeconomic-political context might consider income and social protections; education; unemployment and job insecurity; working life conditions; social inclusion; and, access to affordable health services of decent quality. Within this framework, policy is especially emphasized with attention to the ways in which policies and political movements guide how societies distribute material resources among its citizens and thereby influence persistent health inequities.

In support of the necessity of a consideration of SDOH in health care, the WHO commission provides an example of the inequities in mortality rates noticeable among populations of similar ethnicities. Interestingly, although not surprisingly, are disparities in maternal and child mortality rates of populations residing in poor vs. more affluent neighborhoods that cannot be explained by biology but rather by their social environments. Poverty, however, is not necessarily indicative of poor outcomes. According to research conducted globally, populations with access to increased wealth do not necessarily experience increased health outcomes. Moreover, there is an overreliance on health care systems to address health inequities and less attention to determinants from one's social environment. In order to decrease disparities in mortality rates, a focus on the improvement of daily living conditions is necessary.

The CSDH model has been used to guide the curriculum in a School of Medicine which has included the domains necessary in the education of health professionals (education, community collaboration, and institutional alignment) but also content relevant to a medical school curriculum (racism, discrimination and stigma, poverty, built environment, and access to care) [3, 4]. Reviews of this framework for education suggest the CSDH has utility for curricular guidance or implementation, particularly, with teaching courses focused on community engagement or clinical learning [5, 6].

The Centers for Disease Control (CDC) and Healthy People 2030 Framework Leading organizations have also recognized the importance of SDOH in the health of global populations and have posited a framework with five key areas that focus on: (1) *Access to health care*, (2) *Education access and quality*, (3) *Social and Community Context*, (4) *Economic Stability*, and (5) *Neighborhood and Built Environment* [7] (Fig. 2.2). These five key areas of SDOH have been used to guide a number of research programs through public health through the promotion of safe housing, quality education, and improvements to transportation through community partnerships. Of particular note is the focus on urban geographical locations. Perhaps the more familiar SDOH domain addresses the influences of Access to Health care services to healthy communities—i.e., access to primary health care services, health care insurance, and health literacy. The second domain addresses Education and considers graduation rates from high school, enrollment into college, trade school, or professional schools, as well as access to quality childhood education. The third domain is in the realm of Social and Community Context, that is, community connectedness, civic participation, incarceration, and workplace safety. Fourth, Economic Stability addresses the financial resources available to individuals such as income, cost of living, and one's socioeconomic status which are determinants of health outcomes. Lastly, Neighborhood and Built Environment relate to safe housing, clean air and water, healthy foods, and communities free of crime and violence.

The Socio-Ecological Framework is another frequently cited framework used among schools of public health in the examination of SDOH on health outcomes. The Socio-Ecological Framework is multileveled and considers the complex

Fig. 2.2 Healthy people
SDOH framework

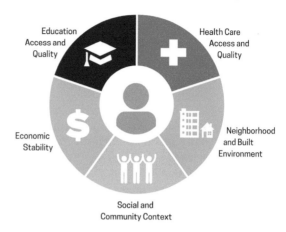

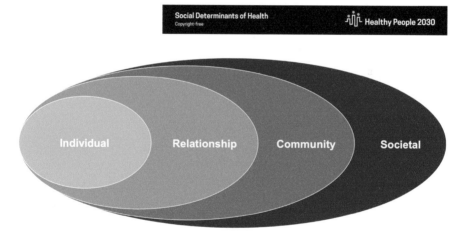

Fig. 2.3 Social-ecological model

interactions among Individual, Relationship, Community, and Societal Levels as a
guide to prevent the excessive burden of illness and mortality rates among populations (Fig. 2.3).

One version of the Social-Ecological framework is also used by the CDC to
guide the development of strategies for the prevention of violence (CDC). The CDC
Social-Ecological Framework used by the CDC includes four levels with consideration for "the complex interplay between individual, relationship, community, and
societal factors," an approach believed more likely to sustain prevention efforts
over time.

The *Individual level* factors consider biological and personal history factors such
as age, income, education, substance use, or history of abuse. *Relationship level*

factors consider close relationships that may increase the risk for violence—i.e., parent/child communication, peer norms, or problem-solving skills. *Community-level* factors consider the settings (schools, workplaces, and neighborhoods) in which social relationships develop and give rise to conditions that promote violence. Finally, *Societal level* factors consider a broad range of determinants that are protective of or encourage violence—i.e., social norms, health, economic, educational, or social policies.

Another version of the Social-Ecological Framework posits four domains and five levels (Fig. 2.4). The four domains include (1) *Socioeconomic Factors* (i.e., education, job status, family/social support, income, and community safety); (2) *Physical Environment*; (3) *Health Behaviors* (tobacco use, diet and exercise, alcohol use, and sexual activity; and (4) *Health care* (access to care and quality of care). At the core of this framework is the belief that SDOHs are complex and interactive factors operating at five levels that include (1) *Individual*, (2) *Interpersonal*, (3) *Organizational*, (4) *Environmental*, and (5) *Public Policy* [8].

The environmental and personal attributes of Social-Ecological Frameworks are consistent with those put forth by public health agencies such as WHO and CDC. The complexity of factors at the individual, community, and societal levels intermingle to protect individuals or place them at risk for illness or premature mortality. In research, the socio-ecological framework has been used as an organizing framework to examine the intersectionality of SDOH conditions such as access to

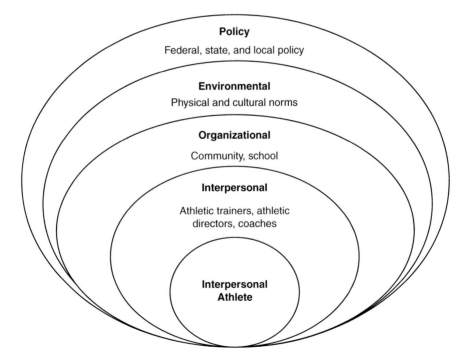

Fig. 2.4 Social-ecological framework

safe housing and food operating at the individual, community, and societal levels to affect chronic disease outcomes [9]. In a study focused on the identification of SDOH factors contributing to physical inactivity, a socio-ecological framework enabled researchers to conclude that an environment of green space and air pollution was important to pleasurable walking [10]. The Socio-Ecological Framework that focuses on the complex interplay of social conditions, environmental conditions, and health behaviors at multilevel influences of individual, community, and societal levels permits the exploration of those SDOH conditions that emerge as the more important influences representative of real-life experiences of populations.

The NIMHD Research Framework is a fourth framework we reviewed for its' utility to guide the integration of SDOH into a nursing curriculum (Fig. 2.5). The NIMHD Framework is a multidimensional model that details domains and levels of influence relevant to understanding and addressing minority health and health disparities. This model guides an examination of Domains at the Individual Level (Behavioral and Sociocultural Environment) and Levels of Influence (Community) [11]. Specifically, the NIMHD Framework can be an organizing framework in our pedagogical efforts to incorporate SDOH content that influences health outcomes among the patients and communities we serve. For example, this NIMHD Framework could be instrumental in the integration of content related to domains that are inclusive of *Biological* factors (the gut microbiome or genetics); *Behavioral* factors (coping strategies, social interactions, or policies and laws; *Physical/Built Environment* inclusive of one's social environment (home, work, school),

National Institute on Minority Health and Health Disparities Research Framework

		Levels of Influence*			
		Individual	Interpersonal	Community	Societal
Domains of Influence (Over the Lifecourse)	**Biological**	Biological Vulnerability and Mechanisms	Caregiver–Child Interaction Family Microbiome	Community Illness Exposure Herd Immunity	Sanitation Immunization Pathogen Exposure
	Behavioral	Health Behaviors Coping Strategies	Family Functioning School/Work Functioning	Community Functioning	Policies and Laws
	Physical/Built Environment	Personal Environment	Household Environment School/Work Environment	Community Environment Community Resources	Societal Structure
	Sociocultural Environment	Sociodemographics Limited English Cultural Identity Response to Discrimination	Social Networks Family/Peer Norms Interpersonal Discrimination	Community Norms Local Structural Discrimination	Social Norms Societal Structural Discrimination
	Health Care System	Insurance Coverage Health Literacy Treatment Preferences	Patient–Clinician Relationship Medical Decision-Making	Availability of Services Safety Net Services	Quality of Care Health Care Policies
Health Outcomes		Individual Health	Family/ Organizational Health	Community Health	Population Health

National Institute on Minority Health and Health Disparities, 2018
*Health Disparity Populations: Race/Ethnicity, Low SES, Rural, Sexual and Gender Minority
Other Fundamental Characteristics: Sex and Gender, Disability, Geographic Region

Fig. 2.5 NIMHD research framework

community resources, and structural determinants; *Sociocultural Environment* (cultural identity, social networks, community and social norms, and structural discrimination; and *Health care* (health literacy, insured status, decision-making, health care policies, and quality of care among levels of influence at the individual, family, community, and societal levels.

Summary of Review of SDOH Frameworks

The frameworks discussed in this chapter are only a few of those that have been in existence for a while or have emerged in response to the recent surge of interest in SDOH. Our critique of these frameworks is solely related to their utility in guiding the integration of SDOH into a school of nursing curriculum. Specifically, these SDOH frameworks suggest domains of influence, levels of influence, and mechanisms by which SDOH content influences health disparities and health inequities. However, we decided to develop a new SDOH for reasons detailed below:

1. A new framework was needed that would be pragmatic for clinical and didactic classroom learning experiences, one that would be easily understood by a nursing faculty with a range of educational backgrounds. Very early in our efforts to integrate SDOH into the curriculum, our faculty clearly articulated their confusion with the many SDOH conceptualizations and even more confusion with existing SDOH frameworks. Frameworks that are complex and focused solely on preventative care would have limited utility for our purpose of SDOH integration throughout the entire curriculum.

    There was a clear need for a framework that could be easily understood and translated into courses beyond population health and rapidly integrated into didactic and clinical courses—even our courses traditionally focused on pathophysiology, pharmacology, and simulation.

2. The discipline of nursing focuses on the delivery of holistic care among populations at varying points of one's life course and at varying points in one's wellness trajectory. Existing SDOH frameworks appear to be developed for the mission and goals of specific disciplines such as Public Health and Medicine and their quest to alleviate preventative illness and enhance access to health care. Our goal was to develop a SDOH framework that would have utility in the promotion of health outcomes and holistic care across acute and chronic health care settings, in urban and rural communities, and among a broad range of ages of patient populations we serve.

3. We also wanted a SDOH framework that would guide faculty and students to consider a broad range of social determinants likely to influence health inequities among diverse populations. The determinants emphasized in the frameworks reviewed appear limited to social and environmental conditions such as access to care, financial constraints, and healthy neighborhoods and among specific populations such as maternal and childcare, urban or adolescent populations. As nursing professionals, we are charged with the delivery of care for a diverse population that extends from the beginning of life to the end of life; at any phase of an illness trajectory; and, the delivery of care in a range of settings.

The Nell Hodgson Woodruff School of Nursing Social Determinants of Health Framework

The Emory School of Nursing Framework is a Four-Pillar approach to integration of SDOH content into the curriculum (Fig. 2.6). This framework pulls content from those SDOH frameworks frequently cited with a consideration for the many social-cultural determinants not easily measured. Our SDOH framework consists of four pillars of social determinants—*Social, Cultural, Environment (physical and social),*

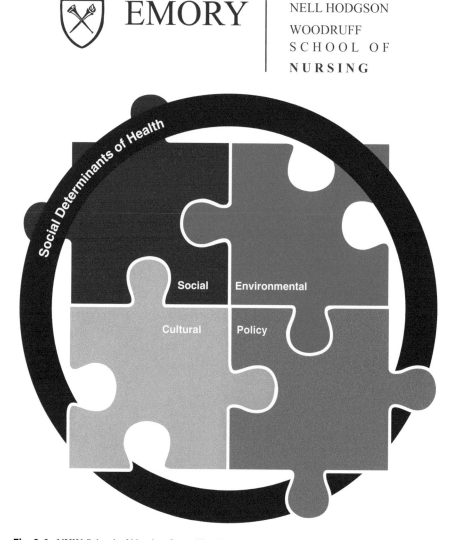

Fig. 2.6 NHW School of Nursing four-pillar SDOH framework

and Policy and is illustrated using interwoven puzzle pieces. This illustration depicts the real-life experiences of individuals that at any given time, these four determinants impact health outcomes. Although one pillar may emerge and be prominent in the promotion of health or alleviation of disease, an imbalance in one is likely to influence the other three SDOH pillars. It is important to consider that at any given time, any one or more of these four pillars can be protective or place individuals at risk for illness and health inequities. In the next sections, we describe each of the four SDOH Pillars with exemplars drawn from research on Americans of African descent. This population is used for exemplars of each SDOH Pillar given the persistent disparities in morbidity and mortality rates experienced among this population.

Social Conditions

Social Conditions are those factors that occur in society due to systemic (structural) racism and imbalances in power, financial resources, education, and occupation that influence wellness or lack thereof (Fig. 2.7). Social conditions shaped by power imbalances and systemic racism for consideration include:

- Access to financial resources, education, type of occupation
- Health literacy
- Access to health care
- Social Support as a Social Resource

Fig. 2.7 Social conditions

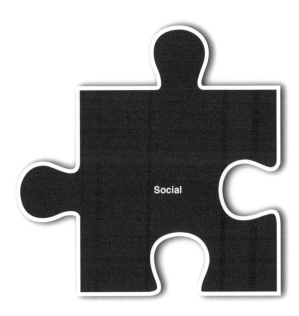

Systemic Racism, Power Imbalance, and Social Conditions

The experience of racism can be from structural and/or interpersonal practices, policies, and social norms that marginalize and oppress individuals or populations based on physical appearances or other visible characteristics. Racism in health care results in the advantage of some populations over others that negatively affects the physical and mental health outcomes of those less advantaged. *Power imbalance* is interwoven with racism and occurs when one group asserts power or dominates another group in ways that disadvantage or are not in the best interest of the other group. *Systemic (structural) racism* and *the imbalance of power* in society are the current focus of educators and health care practitioners in their attempts to understand and dismantle SDOH and health inequities among people of color. Referred to as a major driver of health inequities, systemic racism generally refers to a system of ideas and policies that operate to oppress or marginalize subgroups of its population; a system of beliefs that one group is inherently inferior to another [12]. This type of far-reaching determinant is a widely known and recognized determinant that continues to limit minority groups' access to opportunities and movement from lower stratifications of social classes. Systemic racism has historically limited the ability of people of color to obtain (1) *Financial resources—high-paying jobs with private insurance*, (2) *a quality education*, and (3) *access to quality health care*.

Historical Context of Systemic Racism and Social Conditions

Perhaps the greater illustration of the impact of systemic racism on the interrelatedness of *financial resources (insurance and high-paying jobs), education, and access to health care* can be learned from the history of the enslaved African in the US Historical records dating back to the nineteenth-century documents the poor health outcomes among African Americans that resulted from a system of laws and policies (widely known as Jim Crow Laws) that supported a legal segregation system and also restricted access to health care [13, 14]. During the nineteenth century, systemic racist policies and practices contributed to disproportionately high rates of preventable illnesses such as pneumonia, pellagra, tuberculosis, and syphilis that led to some of the highest rates of premature mortality in the USA [15]. In fact, at the turn of the twentieth century, the life expectancy for these former enslaved Americans was 32 years in comparison to 49 years for white Americans [16]. This racial disparity in mortality rates has been largely attributed to the levels of poverty prevalent among unskilled and skilled occupations and the lack of access to quality education during that time [13, 17].

Employment in low-paying occupations on poor health outcomes among formerly enslaved Americans was especially apparent during the Civil Rights Era [18]. As a result of occupying the lowest income strata, premature mortality rates among this subgroup of Americans continued to be especially high. Even with the integration that occurred during this historical era, access to health care continued to be dismal. In addition to the excessive morbidity rates from deadly illnesses such as cancer, heart disease, and stroke, over one-half of the nation's maternal deaths were among African American women, and the highest infant mortality rates were among African Americans. Persistent racism in the health care system resulted in access to health care that was determined by a person's race but also social class. Even with more advanced cases of cancer and coronary artery disease, African Americans continued to have less access to health care compared to white Americans.

Access to a Quality Education has historically been out of reach for a majority of Americans of African descent. During segregation, for example, African Americans were discouraged from continuing their education beyond what was necessary for employment in service sectors such as domestic or laborers [19]. Reportedly, while white employers were encouraging their descendants and white employees to attend college, they would communicate to their African American employees that they did not need a college education. Inequities in obtaining a quality education were also apparent from the quality of textbooks available to schools in low-income African American communities. Textbooks in schools in communities of color were reportedly discarded from white schools and with pages missing [20]. During the early and mid-twentieth century years, African Americans, for example, grew up attending racially segregated schools and were transported to segregated high schools in a different city (if at all), even when a white school might have been in closer proximity [20]. Although a few partici- pants managed to complete high school during this time, their ability to attend college was hampered by work obligations necessary to assist the family with finances. The experience of African Americans in these segregated schools may have been characterized by education with less experienced or less qualified teachers, high levels of teacher turnover, less successful peer groups, and inade- quate facilities and learning materials than that available to students in majority white schools.

Access to health care facilities expanded during the twentieth century but was still out of reach for many Americans, especially low-income and African Americans. For example, although child health programs were increasingly being established, these programs still were not accessible to the many African Americans in dire need of their services. This increase in access to health care programs during this time was likely a major influence in the improvements in the life expectancy of African American males and females (47 and 49 years, respectively) but was still substan- tially less than that for white Americans (59 years for males and 62 years for females) [15]. For example, while the average life expectancy had increased for both populations since the turn of the century, the gap between the groups had wid- ened from a previous estimate of 5–7 years to 12–13 years [15]. The availability of government-sponsored insurance plans (e.g., Medicaid and Medicare) at least pro- vided payment for some services as these participants became eligible which was believed to increase access to care. However, given the life expectancy of individu- als born in the 1920s and 1930s, it is unlikely that many African Americans lived to the age of 65 years when they would be eligible.

Current and Persistent Social Influences on Health Inequities

Financial resources continue to be a risk factor for disease and mortality rates. The lack of financial resources is often associated with a lack of information and knowledge and timely access to health care when diagnosed with life-threatening illness [21]. For example, persistent white-black disparities among cancer patients have been attributed to lower rates of timely follow-up care after abnormal mammograms and scheduling follow-up appointments which subsequently leads to delays in treatment [21]. And, despite advances in cancer diagnosing and treatment, individuals of a lower SES status (most often identified as racial minorities) are among those with the highest cancer mortality rates [22, 23]. When there is heart disease, the low SES individual is also at risk for higher levels of morbidity and mortality. In at least one national survey, patients with congenital heart disease who identified as Black, of a lower SES (including income and educational levels) had a greater likelihood of death [24]. Similarly, education and income are also determinants of poor hospital outcomes in research among stroke patients [25]. That is, stroke patients with a higher SES (income and educational levels) had low mortality rates while those patients with a low SES (income and education) had high mortality rates [25].

Quality education is more accessible today, however, low educational attainment continues to be a marker for socioeconomic status and resulting higher mortality rates [26]. African Americans are still confronted with the harsh realities of structural racism and the racial segregation that persists among our educational and health care institutions. Older African Americans that lived prior to the Civil Rights Era would likely be disappointed—that is, in spite of the change in laws prohibiting segregation, school segregation is on the rise in the USA. Even in diverse schools, within-school segregation exists where Black, Indigenous, and Latinx adolescents are likely tracked into less rigorous courses and long-term outcomes are likely detrimental to mental health that persists through adulthood [27].

Health literacy is associated with low levels of education and SES status [28]. When patients are not able to understand written information related to their illness, they are less likely to ask questions or to be engaged in their care. For example, in a study examining the association of health literacy on health outcomes among patients with Type 2 diabetes, low levels of health literacy was associated with limitations with medication adherence, depressed moods, and self-management [29]. However, this finding is not consistent. In another study, African American patients with low incomes and health literacy levels were less engaged in behaviors known to lead to better health outcomes [30].

Racial inequities in health care access have persisted into the twenty-first century [31]. Disparate health outcomes have been attributed to poor health behaviors such as lack of exercise, eating fatty foods, and cigarette smoking. However, public health experts and health care practitioners are now acknowledging the powerful influence of structural racism or those influences beyond the control of the individual [32]. Structural inequities such as poverty, the scarcity of health care providers in rural townships, and low-paying jobs without insurance continue to contribute to the limited access to care among low-income and African Americans today [33].

Social Support as a Resource from Family and Friends

Social support from family and friends is generally perceived as a social or financial resource for achieving and maintaining levels of wellness. The most widely known form of social support is emotional support which is the expression of love, liking, or both, and listening to worries and concerns. As a social resource, emotional support might also be in the form of expressions from others that result in feelings of being valued, esteemed, and positive feedback about one's self-worth. Instrumental support is the social resource of material aid or assistance with finances, household tasks, goods and services. The third type of social support, and less frequently studied, is the support from information or advice about some problem or illness.

As a social resource, or SDOH, the availability of social support can be protective or place an individual at risk for poor health outcomes. For many years, the assumption was that social support available to individuals with chronic and life-threatening illnesses was only available among white middle-class and college-educated women; a type of social support not available to lower-income persons and women of color. Scholars have concluded that white and married women were generally among those with higher levels of social support. That is, the support of having someone to confide in about personal and illness concerns among family and friends and to subsequently have an improved outlook on life, better physical functioning, and less likely to have premature mortality rates [34]. The perception that low income and persons of color lack social support is likely influenced by a pattern of research that was conducted primarily among the white middle class and by scientists of similar racial/ethnic backgrounds.

Systemic Racism and Social Support In response to harsh and oppressive living conditions, former enslaved Americans adapted their previous knowledge of family. Family was a system whereby individuals cared for one another and shared available social and financial resources in spite of blood kinship. Even among the lowest of paid workers where there was little or no money, historical accounts of former enslaved Americans document ways in which they shared material resources that enabled their survival—albeit a poor one [17].

Exemplars of the ways in which social support was a resource for low income and persons of color can be examined from narrative accounts during the Great Depression [35]. The Great Depression was difficult for all races/ethnicities, but was particularly devastating for African Americans. Poverty for African Americans was so severe in some situations that there was often little or no money for physical necessities [17, 36]. In situations where there was a lack of money, the support from family and close friends was extremely important to the survival of the African American family; a source of mutual assistance as members shared or bartered services for food, shelter, and clothing [17].

Recent evidence suggests that a lack of social support among African Americans is likely the result of differences in the types of social resources available and utilized among African Americans in comparison to whites. For example, in spite of having very similar health problems, African Americans are less likely to utilize confiding support or be willing to express feelings to others about their problems [37]. The reluctance to confide in others about illness-related problems is related to a fear that one's illness will be a direct burden on family and friends [34]. In fact, the value of not asking for help during times of crisis might be the norm for many members of this population as they are likely to value being perceived as being strong during adverse situations [38]. Emotional support among this population might be expressed through material forms of social support or an emotional presence such as "sitting with the sick" [39], assistance to maintain important social roles at home, church, and work, and sharing stories of hope [37, 40, 41].

Current Influences of Social Support on Health Inequities A culmination of risk factors among African Americans places them among populations most likely to encounter challenges with family support during illness. In comparison to other racial/ethnic groups, African Americans continue to rank lowest with home ownership and are least likely to receive inheritances, gifts, and other financial family support, types of generational wealth that have contributed to better health outcomes among other populations for generations [42]. Additionally, in comparison to white Americans, African Americans are least likely to have recovered from generations of inequities in the job market or even the most recent financial devastation of the Great Recession [42]. The lack of financial resources coupled with generations of limited access to health care services has shaped patterns of giving and receiving social support such that patients are reluctant to ask for help when sick for fear of being a burden to family and friends. Indeed, this perception of being a burden is likely accurate given the harsh realities of limited financial resources in addition to a greater severity of illness and mortality rates experienced.

Inequities in the receipt of social support during illness are especially apparent among African Americans when there is a cancer diagnosis. African Americans continue to experience the highest overall mortality rates, more advanced staged cancers [43], and higher levels of psychological distress from cancer than non-Hispanic Whites [44]. High levels of psychological distress have been linked to unmet needs for support from family and friends and information from health care providers [45]. The root causes of this high level of psychological distress are from a history of past experiences of suffering, death, and isolation witnessed among cancer patients who likely did not survive treatment [41, 43, 46, 47]. African American cancer patients and family members frequently recall images and horror stories of African American cancer patients who "suffered and died," after a period of "wasting away" and in excruciating pain [41]. The stories available to patients and family members are often replete with memories of other cancer patients diagnosed at a late stage and subsequently died from a disease that had spread to the point where treatment would not be effective [41, 47]. Despite high levels of psychological distress, African American patients and family members are not likely to seek mental health services [48] or to participate in hospital-based support groups [49]. African Americans are, however, more likely to participate in community or faith-based support groups as these groups are sensitive to the values and need to remain hopeful and optimistic in the context of life-threatening illness.

Summary of Social Conditions Pillar
In this Social Conditions Pillar, we have covered, at least to some extent, the ways in which the social conditions of financial resources, quality education, type of occupation, health literacy, and access to care as SDOH influence health outcomes. The influence of social conditions on health disparities is especially evident among African Americans, a US population that continues to experience greater health inequities within the context of systemic racism. Other related social factors will be discussed in other SDOH Pillars, i.e., physical environment (safe neighborhoods, access to healthy foods, parks, and recreation areas), and social environment (social integration, support from faith-based institutions).

Cultural Conditions

Cultural conditions are those customary beliefs, social norms, attitudes, values, and practices shared by a group of people (community or society) in a place and time (Fig. 2.8). Cultural conditions shaped by power imbalances and systemic racism for consideration include:

- Interpersonal racism/discrimination
- Religion/spirituality (individual/family values, beliefs)
- Racial memories
- Social norms

Fig. 2.8 Cultural conditions

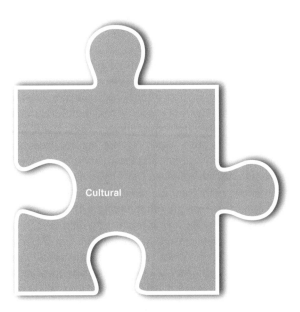

Interpersonal racism/discrimination occurs among one-on-one social interactions, can be negative treatment based on an individual's characteristics, is more identifiable, and likely based on personal beliefs of one group toward another group. In a survey conducted by the Pew Research Center, a majority of African American adults (71%) reported having experienced racial discrimination at some point in their lives from interactions that occurred at the individual level [50]. It has been estimated that during the course of a year, 50% of African American adults report being suspected of wrongdoing (47%), considered as not smart (45%), experiencing unfair treatment in hiring or promotion opportunities (21%), or encountering racial profiling by police (18%) [50]. Although experiences with racism are likely common among African Americans, individuals at greatest risk include men, young adults, and those with some college education. Americans of African descent have consistently reported harsh treatment from the very health care providers in charge of their care when they are most vulnerable [51]. Health care practitioners have a long history of interpersonal racism with formerly enslaved individuals. The medical mistreatment of African Americans is well known, including the racism encountered with the Tuskegee Study, medical experimentation on the vulnerable, and the nonverbal communication that low-income and folk of color were to blame for their poor health [52, 53]. When seeking care from physicians, African Americans have reported an insensitive nature in their communications and this has included spending less time with this population, and lack of respect and warmth during clinic visits [53].

Religion and Spirituality have emerged as powerful determinants of health among US and global populations. Religion is conceptualized as an adherence to a set of beliefs, values, and rituals, and symbols and participation in practices supported by organized faith-based institutions. Religiosity or religious involvement is another concept used among scholars to refer to beliefs and practices related to organized religious institutions [54]. The evidence to support the relationship of religious attendance to higher mortality rates is established. For example, in national surveys, respondents who attend church frequently have a lower hazard of mortality [55].

Spirituality, on the other hand, occurs on a more personal level and apart from affiliations with organized religious institutions. Conceptualizations of spirituality may include a search for answers to questions about life, a relationship to God, and making meaning of individual human experience through dimensions of connectedness: within oneself; to others and the environment; or, to God or other higher power [56]. Conceptualized as the religious practice of praying, spirituality is associated with cognitive functioning and depression [57].

Again, we look to the African American experience to illuminate the ways in which Religion/Spirituality might be protective and/or place the individual at risk for poor health. African Americans are the most religious group in the USA as evidenced by their religious affiliations, engagement in religious practices, and the frequency with which they believe that God exists [58]. Historically, a strong religious culture has been a widely recognized protective factor in illness situations and has enabled African Americans to survive generations of oppression and racism

[59]. In comparison to other racial/ethnic groups, African Americans are more likely to rely on religious beliefs and practices in response to daily life challenges [58]. These religious beliefs and practices have been transmitted through African American oral history and subsequently are closely intermingled with everyday life [59]. As such, they are an important part of African American culture and sources of strength and comfort when confronted with social, personal, and mental health issues.

The practice of using faith-based strategies in response to experienced racial discrimination among African Americans is consistent with a strong religious culture that is generationally influenced [60]. Faith-based strategies may include finding meaning and purpose in the experience or turning to God for support and guidance [61]. Faith-based strategies promote a sense of resilience that buffers the impact of experienced racism on psychological and emotional well-being [62, 63]. A strong religious culture has historically existed among formerly enslaved Americans which has provided individuals with a sense of order and control over their illness. This strong religious culture also promotes self-management of side effects from medical treatments and illness. For example, the survival of the African slave in the USA largely depended on the use of religious songs or memorized scripture passages to communicate their struggles and fears to God and used to encourage one another in during adverse and life-threatening situations [64]. Scholars who have studied the content and purpose of religious songs have determined that these songs consist of Bible-based stories of God delivering oppressed or enslaved persons [65], expressions of the hopes of being delivered from a lifetime of evil and suffering to a lifetime of joy and happiness in this world or the next [65–68].

Religion and spirituality continue to be social determinants among individuals with life-threatening illnesses, particularly among low income and folk of color [69]. The evidence suggests that in comparison to whites, African Americans pray more, and this practice has promoted a more positive attitude toward their cancer experience [70, 71]. In my own research with African Americans, religious beliefs and practices have been used to cope with the loneliness and fears that frequently accompany the cancer experience but to also positively influence the utilization of cancer care services [69]. For example, African American cancer patients have reported praying to God and trusting Him to intercede on their behalf with their worries and providing guidance with treatment-related decisions [72, 73]. A faith in God has been used among recently diagnosed African American cancer survivors to overcome their fears and fatalistic attitudes of cancer being a death sentence and undergo prescribed cancer treatment [74]. A higher level of faith in God and use of religious practices among African American cancer survivors also minimizes treatment side effects, which likely also promotes adherence to treatment [75].

Negative aspects of religion and spirituality are certainly a possibility and are associated with poor health outcomes. Fatalism, a pessimistic perspective, might also occur when patients are blamed and told that their illness is the result of a weakened or lack of faith in God. Rather than religion/spirituality being perceived as a source of comfort, individuals may become distressed with thoughts that they need to pray more or are somehow being tested to see if their faith is strong. These negative and fatalistic attitudes and nonadherence to preventative care may occur when patients believe their illness is the result of a punishment for some sinful behavior. A fatalistic attitude might also be associated with a lack of engagement in cancer screenings [76] and depression [77].

Racial Memories are those experiences, beliefs, and general recollections transmitted from one generation to another. Scholars tend to agree that the intergenerational transmission of stories with racial overtones occur as early as childhood, and persist well into adulthood [78]. Racial memories of the harmful effects of racism might be from structural and/or interpersonal practices, policies, and social norms that marginalized and oppressed individuals or populations based on physical appearances or other visible characteristics. Both historical and even recent scholarship highlights the centuries-old negative impact of racism on the lives of African Americans. For example, in their formative years and much of their adulthood years, older African Americans were exposed to racial violence, segregation, and Jim Crow laws that restricted access to public accommodations, educational institutions, stores, and even access to health care [20]. In rural areas of the Southern US, many African Americans supported themselves through work as sharecroppers which was a form of labor exploitation that resulted in families working for little or no pay [17]. Opportunities for work included employment for men as skilled and unskilled laborers and for women in low paying jobs as domestics and seamstresses [17]. However, these types of employment were without the benefit of private health insurance and therefore a significant contributor to the burden of illness and mortality rates among this population.

In the context of life-threatening illnesses such as cancer, African Americans' racial memories include past recollections of times when cancer was an automatic death sentence. Overall cancer mortality rates for African Americans have also exceeded those of other racial/ethnic groups [79]. In the 1960s, the overall 5-year survival rate for African Americans was a mere 27% which likely fueled the racial memory of an African American cancer experience replete with "suffering and death" after a period of "wasting away" and in excruciating pain [80]. And, among a population that values social connectedness, the fear of death and change in appearance as a result of treatment, further fuels the worry and fear among African Americans that too will die or even worse, be isolated and "pitied" when there is a cancer diagnosis [80]. Racial memories may not lead to a reduction in seeking health care when needed but certainly increase the fear of a negative outcome [80].

Social Norms are those accepted behaviors or ways of thinking that are culturally influenced among groups and can be expected responses to adverse situations such as illness. For example, one possible social norm that influences health outcomes among African American populations can be linked to an internalized value of needing to be strong [38]. Self-reliance or the value of needing to be strong in the face of adversity, occurs when individuals have a preference of relying on their own inner resources. Therefore, help from others is not needed or accepted. The value of self-reliance among an African American population could be attributed to a cultural attitude about asking for help. In a study with older persons of African ancestry (African Americans, Afro-Barbadians, and Afro-Haitians), participants believed they should give help but not ask for help in return [81]. In a study of low-income African American women, 15% said they never call on friends or relatives for help with health problems, rather they tend to rely only on themselves [82].

Another social norm that occurs among African Americans is to not openly discuss certain illnesses. Mental illness, for example, is associated with a stigma that results in a significant problem among African American populations [83–85]. African Americans are 20% more likely than whites to report serious psychological distress [86], fear public prejudice and discrimination [85, 87], and to be misdiagnosed by health care providers [85], African Americans also report being fearful of being labeled "crazy" within their families and communities when there is mental illness [88]. Although the precise origins of this mental illness stigma are less clear, there is general agreement that stigma results in a higher illness burden among African Americans [87, 89]. High levels of psychological distress require appropriate health care, however, mental health care providers skilled at delivering culturally competent care are limited and Americans of African descent are also more likely to turn to forms of religious coping such as prayer and a belief in God [85, 90].

Summary of Cultural Conditions Pillar

In this Cultural Conditions Pillar, we have covered, at least to some extent, the ways in which the cultural conditions of interpersonal racism/discrimination, religious beliefs, spirituality, racial memories as SDOH influence health outcomes and health equities among former enslaved US population. Depending on the population, other cultural conditions important for consideration might include societal values and nursing values. Although these cultural conditions have been discussed somewhat in this chapter among African Americans of a protestant religious tradition, further consideration might include the ways in which social norms or informal rules exist among patients from varied cultures and other religious traditions.

Environmental (Physical) Conditions (Part I)

Physical—the part of the human environment that includes purely physical factors (Fig. 2.9). Physical environmental conditions for consideration include:

- Natural Resources/Natural Disasters
- Climate Change/extremes in heat and cold temperatures
- Exposure to toxic substances
- Recreational resources—Safe play spaces

Historical Overview of Nursing and Environmental Health Threats Nursing has a long history of responding to threats to health from disruptions in the environment. Dating back to Florence Nightingale, nurses have stepped into global or national leadership roles in response to environmental hazards that have threatened the lives of families and the communities in which they lived [91]. In the nineteenth

Fig. 2.9 Physical
environmental conditions

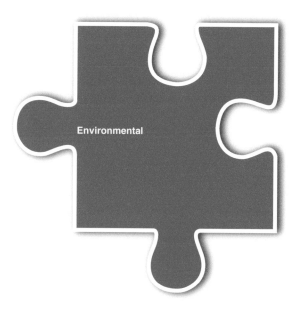

and early twentieth centuries, housing and labor protections were in their infancy and primarily focused on shoddy construction sites, substandard sanitation systems, abusive landlords, and poor urban planning [91]. Around the mid-twentieth century, patient care transitioned from community to hospital settings, when the focus of care shifted less attention was directed to risk factors for disease [91]. Care in hospital settings encouraged nurses to focus on sick-patient care among patients with specific illness; a shift from a holistic approach to care [91]. This shift to sick-patient care also fostered a perspective of care that is now largely focused on optimizing care rather than optimizing an environment that is healthy.

Several other historical events in the twentieth century shifted the perception of environmental issues being isolated events to those more widespread social issues. These social issues have included military troops' exposure to Agent Orange abroad and devastating community exposure to pollutants in the homeland. For example, the 1956 "Smog Complex" caused more than 2000 traffic accidents in the city of Los Angeles, California in just 1 day [91]. Another environmental threat of great magnitude was the devastation from wastewater and industrial runoff that contaminated farm soil and water supplies that disproportionately affected low-income and minority communities [91]. Environmental threats have been from rivers and lakes that have been so riddled with sewage, oil, and industrial runoff, like the Cuyahoga River in 1969, that the pollutants caught fire and resulted in the deaths of countless wildlife [91].

In the next sections, we highlight a few determinants related to physical and social environmental conditions. As with the social and cultural determinants, we illustrate environmental conditions using the evidence from populations most affected; low income and African Americans.

Natural Resources/Natural Disasters Poverty and/or racism has influenced the severity of the impact of natural disasters on individuals, communities, and societies. Natural disasters can affect anyone at any given time, the long-term impact of flooding from hurricanes and extremes in temperature disproportionately affects residents of low-income communities globally. In the USA, systemic racism has led to an inadequate infrastructure in some cities that fails to protect its low-income citizens. Poverty guarantees that the financial resources of some individuals will only get worse during natural disasters. Perhaps one of the most devastating encounters from a natural disaster occurred over a decade ago that disproportionately affected low-income African Americans in Louisiana during the aftermath of Hurricane Katrina [92]. Hurricane Katrina was a destructive and deadly Category 5 tropical storm that made landfall in Louisiana and Mississippi on August 29, 2005. The flooding in the city of New Orleans in Louisiana has been largely attributed to engineering flaws in the levees (flood protection system constructed by the US government) around the city [92]. Residents of this city with financial resources were able to evacuate before the hurricane made landfall. However, low-income and African Americans were not so fortunate. Those residents without the financial resources to evacuate endured days without water, food, or shelter. Many residents died from thirst, fatigue, and the violence that occurred in shelters. Katrina victims were either displaced from their homes, relocated and separated from family. Those that did return found homes in shambles and uninhabitable.

Climate Change/Extremes in Heat and Cold Temperatures The earth's climate has experienced a change in the atmosphere which has raised the global temperature and extremes in weather patterns [93]. Threats to society from warmer temperatures have been the focus of the Environmental Protection Agency (EPA) for several years. Extremes in the weather have resulted in wildfires, air pollution, and floods. Extreme heat has been linked to illness and deaths, especially among the poor, pregnant women, children, elderly, and migrant farm workers [93, 94]. Climate change is a global issue and known contributor to a rise in cardiovascular disease [95], complications of diabetes [96], asthma mortality rates [97], and increased mortality risk among the elderly [97]. In North America, however, low income and communities of color are especially impacted given the inequitable distribution of resources and social status [94, 98].

Increases in morbidity and mortality rates from environmental threats are predicted for the next several decades. The burden of extremes in weather is expected to be especially high among non-Hispanic Black infants and Australian indigenous infants who are much more likely to be born preterm than other racial/ethnic groups [99]. The increase in premature births among these populations is attributed to racism and classism (lack of access to high-quality care) and community and environmental health (exposure to air pollution, lack of green space, and exposure to violence) [99]. The elderly is another population more likely to be negatively impacted by extremes in heat. Among the elderly and elderly African Americans, extremes in heat are a known contributor to increased Emergency Room (ER) visits for mental health issues [100]. Extremes in heat also contribute to increases in hospitalizations from myocardial infarctions particularly during summer months [101].

Exposure to Toxic Substances Toxic substances are harmful to individual, family, and community health. These include exposure to fumes from cleaning agents, harmful chemicals present in drinking water or foods, air pollutants, and even pesticides used in the production of the foods we eat [102]. Probably one of the more well-known toxins that had widespread harmful health effects was from asbestos exposure. Exposure to asbestos is known to increase the incidence of lung disease so much so that major national initiatives were implemented to ban the use of this substance and mandate its removal from public buildings [102]. Another more recent example of an environmental threat was from toxic substances found in drinking water exposed during the Flint water crisis. The Flint water crisis began when elevated levels of lead were found in children who had been drinking the city's water. Scholars have suggested that this lead-contaminated water disproportionately affected a city that is largely low income and African American. This contaminated drinking water resulted in excessive fetal deaths and other harmful health effects from ingesting lead from a water supply to numerous children during their formative years [103, 104]. Although the state of Michigan installed water filters, replaced pipes, and provided health care, educational and food resources to those affected, residents remain distrustful that the water is truly safe [105]. Moreover, research conducted years later suggests long-term effects leading to depression and post-traumatic distress disorder among adults living in the aftermath of this disaster [105].

Recreational Resources: Safe Play Spaces Access to recreational resources including safe play spaces that permit children and adults to engage in outdoor activities has many benefits. In a community–academic partnership, renovated safe play spaces in schoolyards increased physical activity and social interactions in a low-income, urban neighborhood [106]. Green schoolyards may buffer against the effects of urbanization by increasing access to nature. A renovated green schoolyard has been shown to increase physical activity, schoolyard safety, school–community relationships, and less bullying behaviors [106]. Green schoolyards also offer a safe space for children and adults to engage in social, outdoor activities, particularly in low-income, urban neighborhoods [106]. Additionally, safe and green spaces that incorporate strategies to lower the traffic flow in urban areas decrease unhealthy weight trajectories in children [107].

Although safe green spaces generally encourage outdoor play and social activities, these healthy behaviors were reduced for some populations during the COVID pandemic when youth and adults were physically restrained to their homes [108]. For example, while youths with higher incomes and access to a safe built environment were more active and played more outdoors, low-income and Hispanic minority youth felt less safe [108]. Low-income residents who were older, female, and black engaged in outdoor physical activity even though their neighborhoods were not safe [109].

Summary of Physical Environment
In this section, we discussed some of the prevailing physical environmental threats to human health. Nursing has a long history of identifying and addressing physical environmental threats beginning with a focus on holistic care in communities to sick-patient care in hospital settings. This shift to sick-patient care with specific illness may have contributed to a lack of focus on holistic care, an emphasis on nursing care in previous years. In this section on physical environmental conditions, we have focused our discussion on natural resources/natural disasters, climate change, exposure to toxic substances, and safe play spaces, conditions prevalent in our communities. Although we recognize there are many other threats from the physical environment, we are hopeful that the ones discussed will inspire your thinking on ways to incorporate those of interest to your faculty and students.

Environmental (Social) Conditions (Part II)

Social environment is defined as a social setting in which people live (Fig. 2.10).

Social environment might be further defined as the surroundings (social settings) that are influenced by humans. In this section, we detail a few social settings important to health equity including quality of schools/academic settings, housing, access to affordable transportation, faith-based institutions, quality of schools, and composition of families. Other aspects of social settings important to consider as SDOH would be transportation, safety of neighborhoods, and community design. We have previously discussed access to health care and education. In this section, we consider:

- Quality of schools/academic settings
- Workforce Diversity in Health care
- Housing (safe and quality housing)
- Faith-based institutions
- Composition of families

Quality of Schools, Academic Settings Historically, former enslaved Americans fought to obtain higher educational levels believing this to be the path to equality, independence, and respect [110]. A major triumph in the struggle for a quality education for this population was the passage of the Civil Rights Act of 1964. In the years leading up to the Civil Rights Act, older African Americans recalled attending racially segregated schools and being transported to segregated high schools in a different city, even when a white school might have been in closer proximity [20].

Fig. 2.10 Social environmental conditions

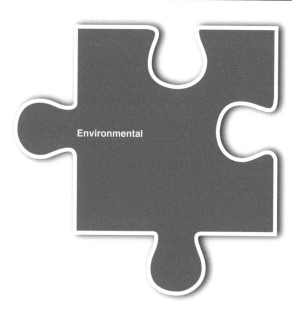

In rural areas, especially this transportation issue prevented many older African Americans from graduating from high school or even attending college. In addition to transportation issues, poverty contributed to unequal access to educational resources. For example, in rural areas and among low-income families, the ability to complete high school and attend college was hampered by work obligations [20]. Poverty often dictated that everyone in the family contribute financially to keep the family housed and fed. Not unheard of are stories of children missing school days for work or teens dropping out of school altogether to enter the workforce [20]. Even when schools were accessible, students in segregated schools in African American communities could have received an inferior education with less experienced or less qualified teachers, high levels of teacher turnover, less successful peer groups, and inadequate facilities and learning materials than exist in majority white schools.

Although there have been gains made in accessing a quality education post-segregation for African Americans, the harsh realities of structural racism and racial segregation persist among our educational institutions. In spite of the change in laws prohibiting segregation, school segregation is on the rise in the USA [111]. Even in schools claiming a diverse student population, within-school segregation exists. Moreover, attaining a quality education continues to be linked to one's social status. Today, the overwhelming majority of African American students attend under sourced schools where a majority of them are also African American [112]. Low-income and African American students in these schools are also likely tracked into less rigorous courses resulting in detrimental long-term outcomes that are detrimental to their health and wellness; outcomes that persist throughout adulthood [27].

Our sickest patients today with the highest mortality rates are those with a low educational level [113].

Health care Workforce Diversity A diverse health care workforce is critical to the delivery of care that is culturally sensitive. Health care is still lacking adequate numbers of providers with the knowledge and skillset necessary for care that is respectful and equitable. Scholars believe this lack of diversity in health care is severe and not likely to change [114, 115]. Historically, a period of racial segregation (Jim Crow) contributed greatly to a lack of hospitals and health care providers within majority African American and rural communities [14, 116]. During segregation, black-owned and run hospitals filled the void in health care, however, due to a lack of funding, hospitals, and clinics in these areas were also of a lower quality than those of majority-white communities and virtually nonexistent today [116]. Even among hospitals that were integrated, African American health care providers were not allowed to practice in these settings, further alienating low-income African Americans from receiving optimal health care [116]. In the twentieth century, hospitals with Magnet status, NCI-Designated Cancer Centers, and Designated Trauma Centers generally provide a higher level of care and are likely to employ a more diverse workforce. However, these medical centers are not easily accessible to populations with limited financial resources and challenges with transportation.

Housing (Safe and Quality Housing) Substandard housing as a SDOH among low income, rural, and African American populations, especially brought to light during the COVID-19 pandemic. Substandard housing interwoven with limited access to health care, and prolonged occupational exposure from this virus was especially noticeable among low-income and residents of rural communities [117]. The impact of substandard housing among these populations has been devastating and particularly noticeable with the excessive mortality rates experienced among rural populations [117]. Even among rural residents, African Americans have been more likely than whites to live in substandard housing, in poverty, and in households headed by women.

Substandard housing is important to health care for several reasons. First, families in communities with substandard housing are less likely to have access to financial resources, quality educational institutions, or even health care than residents living in more affluent neighborhoods. Secondly, residents of substandard housing are at higher risk for poor mental and physical health [118]. The findings of recent research suggest that an overwhelming majority of US households reported one or more subpar housing domain associated with poor health [119]. Prevalent among these domains included household fuel combustion, dampness and mold, inadequate water and sanitation, and injury hazards. Pests and allergens, low indoor temperatures, and injury hazards were consistently associated with older homes, lower rent costs, and lower unit satisfaction [119].

A more troubling issue for impoverished communities of color comes from the persistent violence that occurs among residents in these communities [120]. Communities with substandard housing are also communities with high rates of violence. For example, homicide is the number one killer of young black males while intimate partner violence disproportionately kills black women [120]. These communities are also characterized by gang violence, excessive use of police force, and the rise in suicide rates [120].

Faith-Based Institutions Historically, a primary social institution that promoted the well-being of African Americans has been the Black Church. This faith-based and social institution originated from gatherings of former enslaved Americans as a place where they could exercise their religious beliefs apart from the control of the white slave owners. Although the African slave came to America from many different African tribes and religious backgrounds, historians tend to agree that religion was very important to the survivorship of this population [64, 121, 122]. In fact, historical literature describes the Black church as an "invisible institution" whereby the African slave in America secretly met to worship and express their sorrows to God and to believe in His ability to deliver them from the evils of this world [64]. These expressions were important mental health-promoting strategies that permitted the African slave to express pent-up emotions about their slave experiences and to receive emotional support for their plight through socializing and visiting with family and friends [123].

The Black Church has maintained its role as a major faith-based institution for largely African American congregations. Over time and since slavery, the Black Church has expanded its role from religious service to the promotion of services specifically designed to combat specific health and social problems that disproportionately affect the larger African American community [124–126]. For example, in response to increases in youth crime rates, poor educational systems, and the need for after-school care for working parents, the Black Church has developed educational programs for children [126]. In response to the disproportionate rates of cancer among African Americans, churches have organized large-scale cancer screening programs [127, 128] and cancer support groups [129]. Other ongoing formal support services provided assistance with personal care services and housekeeping and transportation to church, stores, and physician appointments [130].

In recent years, health care providers have partnered with the Black Church to enhance the delivery of health care services in underserved communities. Since the Black Church is generally embedded in underserved communities with long-term trusting relationships, health care providers have effectively delivered the influenza vaccine [131], cancer control interventions [132], COVID information and vaccines [133–136] and cardiovascular mobile health interventions [136].

Compositions of Families/Naturally Occurring Social Interactions and Social Connectedness Extended family generally refers to close familial relationships among people that otherwise would not be included in the traditional nuclear household [124, 137, 138]. McAdoo (1991) described extended family members as close relationships that include persons related by blood or marriage but a unit that often extends to include friends and neighbors who are referred to as fictive kin [126]. The phrase fictive kin is used because these persons are not related by blood but relationships with these persons are so close they are considered to be "like family." The relationships of these persons are so close that they are often referred to as aunt, uncle, cousin, play sister, or brother [138]. Extended family members may consist of family members who reside in the same household or throughout several households.

A dominant thought in American culture is that the traditional family structure consists of a married couple with children. However, the traditional family structure is less likely among African Americans and individuals living in poverty [139]. One prevalent family structure is the single-mother household. Single-mother households are less likely to have completed college and more likely to live in poverty than other family structures. This disparity is especially pronounced among African American women, who in recent years are much more likely to be never married or divorced [139]. African American children in these single-mother households are even more affected—with a majority living in poverty [139].

Scholars studying the African American family have noted that any deviation from the traditional two-parent nuclear family has been negatively criticized and labeled dysfunctional [124, 140]. A predominant stereotype that the African American female-headed household is largely dependent on the welfare system is an erroneous assumption not verified by research. In fact, data show that aid to African American female-headed households from welfare and food stamps accounts for only 28% of the income for these family groups [141]. Moreover, Census Bureau data reveal that, in the time period between 1979 and 1989, the percentage of African American families receiving welfare benefits decreased from 24 to 21% [125]. When researchers focus on negative elements of African American families, such as persons on welfare, they fail to see positive characteristics that exemplify the majority of African American families. For example, although 28% of African American female-headed households receive public welfare, the overwhelming majority, or 72% of these households, are not dependent on welfare as a source of income but self-sufficient, productive members of society [141].

Summary of Social Environmental Conditions

In this social environmental conditions section, we discussed the ways in which social settings were determinants of health inequities. The quality of schools/academic settings, workforce in health care diversity, safe and quality housing, faith-based institutions, and composition of families were discussed. Other social environmental conditions for consideration would be access to public transportation that is convenient and affordable and a discussion on the access to advanced education at quality educational institutions continues to be out of reach for low income and persons of color. Not surprisingly, education that is affordable and of high quality continues to be less accessible to low income and persons of color. The lack of a diverse workforce in health care has been an issue for decades. Health care providers with the skillset to truly understand social and cultural issues of relevance to diverse patient populations are desperately needed, particularly as society becomes more diverse. It is no surprise that substandard housing is influenced by a lack of financial resources and places low-income individuals in unsafe neighborhoods, leading to fears of safety and low levels of physical activity. On the other hand, when individuals have the resources to live in quality houses, safe neighborhoods, health outcomes are improved. Finally, faith-based institutions and the composition of families, especially among African Americans have been a protective influence, a strategy to alleviate situations where there is a lack of financial resources. The Black Church and extended family have historically responded to racism and oppression through community and by sharing what resources were available to them.

Policies/Laws

Guidelines, principles, legislation, and activities that affect the living conditions conducive to the welfare of individuals, communities, and societies quality of life (Fig. 2.11). Policies implemented on a national, regional, or even within institutions at a local level have been protective for some populations and devastating for others. In this section, we discuss a few policies/laws initiated at a national level that has contributed to health outcomes for individuals, families, and communities. In this section we reflect on the following:

- Jim Crow Laws/Civil Rights Act
- Government Sponsored insurance plans
- Abortion (Roe vs. Wade)
- COVID-19 Vaccines

Black Codes and Jim Crow Laws Perhaps the Law with the greater influence on persistent racial disparities in health care originated from Jim Crow Laws that legalized racial segregation for nearly 100 years after the Civil War. Enforced until 1965, Jim Crow laws mandated racial segregation in public institutions in Southern US States [142]. The intent of these laws was to marginalize African Americans through the denial of certain rights—the right to quality education, high-paying jobs, and health care [143]. Interwoven with Jim Crow Laws were Black codes that restricted the rights and freedoms of African Americans [143–145]. Black codes were strictly local and state laws that dictated when and where formerly enslaved Americans could work, where they could live, how they could travel, and whether they could vote [143, 145]. There were also laws that would permit authorities to seize

Fig. 2.11 Policy
conditions

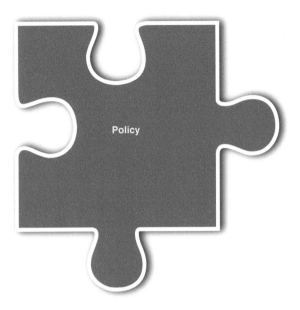

formerly enslaved individuals, including children, for forced labor without pay [142]. Segregation was enforced in neighborhoods, recreation parks, public pools, hospitals, and residential homes for handicapped and disabled individuals [145].

Although *Jim Crow* laws ended in 1968, the effect of racial segregation persists and is a SDOH for descendants of the American slavery system [146]. Jim Crow laws dictated that African Americans attend segregated schools that provided an education that was of a lower quality than that of their white counterparts [143, 145]. In spite of the Brown vs. Board of Education ruling that racial segregation in public schools was unconstitutional, there are reports of continued segregation in public schools today [147]. An inferior education frequently translates into the inability to obtain higher paying jobs with the benefit of private insurance, to obtain housing in safe neighborhoods with better quality schools, financial resources to purchase fresh fruits and vegetables, and greater access to quality health care.

Jim Crow laws have not only had a negative impact on education but are also apparent in the utilization of hospital services and the structure and functioning of minority communities. Moreover, these negative effects have persisted long after these laws ended in 1965 and influence racial disparities in health care today. For example, in comparison to whites, blacks under-utilize primary care and overutilize emergency department services. Health care practitioners have long believed that the underutilization of primary care was the result of distrust. However, recent research presented evidence to suggest that this pattern of health care services use is likely attributed to the ways in which non-Hispanic blacks were socialized during this extended period of racial segregation [148]. That is, the denial of access to health care during segregation contributes to a population's underuse of primary care and seeking care when the illness has advanced to a severe stage. In other research, social capital among residents in the Southern US was found to have persisted after Jim Crow laws were abolished. In comparison to non-Jim Crow states, the effects of racial segregation on lower levels of income, lower social connectedness, and the ability of communities to respond collectively to threats [146].

Government Sponsored Insurance Racism and racial inequities in the delivery of health care have persisted into the twenty-first century [31]. Although disparate health outcomes are attributed to poor health behaviors such as a lack of exercise, fatty foods, and cigarette smoking, public health experts and health care practitioners are now acknowledging the powerful influence of conditions beyond the control of the individual [32]. Poverty, the scarcity of health care providers in rural townships, and low-paying jobs without insurance all contribute to a poor quality of care experienced among African Americans today [149]. The availability of government sponsored insurance plans (e.g., Medicaid and Medicare) at least provided payment for some services as these participants became eligible. However, given the life expectancy of individuals born in the 1920s and 1930s, it is unlikely that many African Americans born during that time period lived to the age of eligibility. Without health insurance and no health care providers in some geographical areas, low income and African Americans were destined for high mortality rates.

Government sponsored insurance plans such as Medicare and Medicaid that came after the Jim Crow years and is thought of as the most important Civil Rights Achievements in US history [150]. The federal government literally threatened to withhold federal funding from hospitals that refused to desegregate [150]. This government sponsored insurance plan forced the desegregation of hospitals benefited African Americans but low income persons as well [150]. In the next sections, we examine advantages and disadvantages of government sponsored insurance plans, particularly among low income and African Americans.

Medicare and Medicaid are the more well-known types of government sponsored insurance programs [151]. Medicare generally covers hospital care for people over the age of 65 years, younger disabled persons, and patients on dialysis [151]. There are no premiums for Medicare Part A (Hospital Insurance) for individuals aged 65 years who are permanent citizens or residents of the USA. Medicare Part A is also available to US citizens under the age of 65 years who, for example, are on dialysis or have had a kidney transplant [151]. Medicare Part B (Medical Insurance) has a premium that is paid either monthly or quarterly. Medicare Part C, referred to as a Medicare Advantage Plan, is offered by private companies approved by Medicare. For an additional premium, Medicare Advantage Plans provide extra coverage for vision, hearing, dental, or health and wellness plans. Medicare Part D is another option that comes with a premium to help cover the cost of prescription medications. Out-of-pocket costs for these Medicare Advantage Plans can vary by the company according to their rules. These plans have rules that set fees for out-of-pocket costs that can change yearly. Medicaid is a health care coverage program for low-income children, adults, pregnant women, seniors, and people with disabilities

[151]. For those individuals who are eligible, Medicaid covers emergency ambulance services, and dental services.

The Affordable Care Act (ACA) is a health insurance coverage available to individuals, families, and small businesses [152]. These insurance plans are operated by individual states and may be used to expand Medicaid coverage to their low-income families and individuals. The ACA was signed into law on March 23, 2010, as the Patient Protection and Affordable Care Act and amended on March 30, 2010, by the Health Care and Education Reconciliation Act. The ACA addresses gaps in health insurance coverage, health care costs, and preventive care among US citizens and residents. The benefit of being insured under the ACA is that health insurance companies cannot refuse to pay for care related to preexisting conditions like other individual insurance policies.

These government sponsored insurance plans were designed to lessen the burden of cost to access to health care among low-income individuals and to decrease health disparities. However, recent scholarship suggests that disparities in accessing health care persist among socioeconomically disadvantaged patients. For example, low-income patients with Medicaid were more likely than private/Medicare patients to be diagnosed with later staged cancers [153, 154]. Low-income women with breast cancer are more likely to have longer travel times to a plastic surgeon and less likely to receive breast construction than other similarly staged women with Medicaid insurance coverage [155]. Still, other research suggests that persons experiencing homelessness, a subpopulation of Medicaid patients, are underutilizing health care services that would be covered under this program [156]. The underutilization of health care services among low-income persons with Medicaid coverage suggests that social factors other than one's ability to pay for services play a role in health outcomes.

Roe vs. Wade   The original Roe v. Wade was a legal case decided by the US Supreme Court on January 22, 1973, that ruled that state regulation of restricting abortions was unconstitutional [157]. The Roe v. Wade opinion stated that in most instances the criminalization of abortion violated a woman's constitutional right to privacy. This was a constitutional right and consistent with a clause of the Fourteenth Amendment that no state shall deprive any person of life, liberty, or property, without due process of law. The 1973 Roe v. Wade decision was based on a federal action against the district attorney of Dallas county, Texas. At that time, the US Supreme Court disagreed that women should have the right to terminate pregnancy in any way and at any time and supported the termination of a pregnancy at approximately the end of the first trimester of pregnancy. In 2022, after many years of discussions and disagreements about the constitutionality of abortions, Roe v. Wade was reversed.

The decision to overturn Roe v. Wade has become extremely controversial and in this chapter we will not argue whether or not women's rights are being violated. Rather, we examine the influence of increased illegal and unsafe abortions on the morbidity and mortality of women that may result from this policy. Scholars have presented evidence that abortions are safe when conducted in a legal setting under safe conditions, however, the general consensus is that the majority of abortions are not conducted under safe conditions [158–160]. According to the World Health Organization (WHO), approximately 45% of all abortions are unsafe and 97% of those occur in developing countries [161]. The WHO has reported that abortions performed under unsafe conditions have contributed to injuries and deaths of women worldwide [161]. Unsafe abortions contribute to 4.7–13.2% of maternal deaths yearly and in 2012 alone, estimates are that seven million women per year were hospitalized for complications from unsafe abortions [161]. Currently, illegal abortions are reportedly much lower in the USA in comparison to women of lower-resourced developing countries [159, 160].

Globally, low-income women bear the greater financial burden of unsafe abortions. There may be costs associated with travel, mandatory waiting periods, or loss of income that limit access to safe abortion care for women with low resources [161]. Unsafe abortions are not only financially burdensome for the women but this burden extends to the family. WHO estimates from 2006 suggest that the cost of unsafe abortions to US households was 922 million in loss of income as a result of long-term disability from unsafe abortions [161]. In comparison, unsafe abortions are significantly higher in countries with highly restrictive abortion laws than in those countries with less restrictive laws [161]. However, when abortions have been legalized and subsidized, the maternal morbidity rates have declined drastically [162].

Coronavirus Disease (COVID-19) and Vaccine Rollout COVID-19 is an infectious disease caused by the SARS—CoV-2 virus which was initially discovered in December 2019 in Wuhan, China. Since that time COVID-19 rapidly spread throughout the world resulting in the deaths of millions. The contagiousness of the COVID-19 virus is due to its ability to replicate inside a cell and quickly spread to other cells. Its ability to constantly mutate has resulted in a virus with variants that are deadly and must be continually monitored [163].

According to the latest COVID-19 statistics, there have been 615 million recorded cases and 6.5 million deaths worldwide [164]. In the USA alone, there have been 95.9 million cases and 1.05 million deaths. COVID-19 also resulted in what is now known as post-COVID (Long COVID) conditions that can occur after COVID-19 infection and include a wide range of ongoing health problems that last weeks, months, and can lead to disability [163]. Individuals at higher risk for post-COVID conditions include those not vaccinated [163].

Information about the COVID-19 virus began to be disseminated in the USA in January 2020 which initially followed with guidelines for physical distancing and wearing masks. However, the news was slow to reach some communities and information that was disseminated was not trusted particularly among those most vulnerable. COVID-19 was especially devastating for the African American community. African Americans have experienced a higher number of COVID-19 cases and hospitalizations than non-Hispanic whites [165]. In fact, COVID-19 mortality rates for

African Americans are a third higher than for Latinos and more than double that for whites [166]. Although we are still in this pandemic, scholars have posited that the stark COVID-19 disparity among African Americans is a result of long existing systemic racist policies. Policies that continue to have lasting effects on access to quality education, financial resources, housing, employment, and access to care [165]. The COVID-19 pandemic brought to light the determinants that prevented many African Americans from adhering to WHO and CDC guidelines for social distancing. Housing, community, and economic status is a privilege that permitted those with resources to adhere to protective guidelines—i.e., the privilege to work from home, to shop online, to buy N95 masks and hand sanitizer. African Americans account for a larger percentage of Americans with low resources—jobs that are low paying and in the service sector and among those who use public transportation which increased their exposure to this community-acquired infection [165].

Despite the CDC's commitment to vaccine equity, access to this antiviral medication has been especially challenging for African American and Latino people and likely contributed to their higher incidence of illness and higher mortality rates from COVID-19 [167]. Scholars have concluded that the low rates of COVID-19 vaccines among African American and Latino populations have been the result of hesitancy or resistance behaviors [168–170]. Hesitancy behaviors have been linked back to mistreatment of African American and Latino communities, distrust of health care, and structural barriers to accessing the vaccine [170].

Although scholars have focused their attention to vaccine hesitancy and mistrust as the contributor to a lack of vaccine uptake, lack of access to the vaccine is likely the greater issue [171, 172]. When the focus of low rates of vaccine uptake has been directed to vaccine hesitancy, scholars and practitioners have not recognized the burden imposed from factors not within the individual's control. Moreover, the latest trends in vaccine hesitancy suggest that in comparison to whites, there has been a recent shift from fewer Black adults with the "wait and see" attitude to higher numbers waiting to get vaccinated [172]. Reports from communities of color suggest that the initial vaccine rollout was not accessible due to structural barriers. One structural barrier included a lack of access to pharmacies or pharmacy services in rural areas or communities of color. Scheduling, computer literacy, transportation difficulties, and computer/Internet access have also been reported as structural barriers that created challenges for persons of color wanting to be vaccinated [172].

The US Census Bureau has reported that among all households in 2018, 92% had a computer, laptop, tablet, or smartphone and 85% had a broadband internet subscription [173]. However, the creation of a vaccine scheduling system that was complex to navigate made it difficult to impossible even for persons with Internet access to schedule an appointment. The initial phases of the vaccine rollout required that eligible persons make an appointment through a system where appointments were often closed out before they could be confirmed. Even when an appointment was confirmed, it was frequently with a government sponsored vaccine center located in another town or city not easily accessible via car or public transportation. Additionally, while many households had Internet connections, Black, Hispanic, and low-income households rely on smartphones and are likely to incur costs should data usage exceed that allowed under specific plans with cell phone providers [173].

A vast majority of US citizens travel by car or use public transportation. However, the American Public Transportation Association (APTA) reports that nearly 42% of Americans have only one car and 45% of Americans still do not have access to public transportation [174]. Initially, travel to government sponsored vaccine centers required access to private or public transportation which limited access for the homebound, elderly, and disabled. Structural barriers from transportation challenges limited access to the vaccine for those at higher risk of contracting and dying from COVID-19.

Other challenges were related to the inconvenience of scheduling for essential employees and immigration status. Essential workers generally include those in health care, food service, transportation, and emergency services [175]. These individuals are among those least likely to have flexibility in their schedules that permits access to the vaccine. Since oftentimes appointments were only available during traditional 9–5 office or clinic hours, both essential workers and immigrants may have had scheduling issues. Immigrants may have also encountered language issues, fears related to immigration enforcement arrests, or fears related to residency status [172].

Summary of Policy Conditions

Although Policy Conditions have not generally been the focus of social determinants of health, this pillar is truly the foundation of the other three Pillars (Social, Cultural, and Environmental) of the Nell Hodgson Woodruff SDOH Framework presented in this chapter. In this chapter on Policy Conditions, we discuss four policies that have shaped health outcomes, particularly, for low-income and African American populations. Jim Crow laws that ended in 1968 legalized racial segregation in public spaces in the Southern US. However, these years of racial segregation have had long-lasting effects on inequities in education, income, wealth, home ownership, and even the type of occupation available to descendants of former enslaved Americans. In spite of widespread integration in public spaces, schools and neighborhoods remain segregated. We also discuss three other controversial policies implemented at the national level: Affordable Care Act, Roe v. Wade, and the rollout of the COVID-19 vaccine. Even though policies were intended to have equitable benefit to all persons, evidence suggests that low-income and persons of color with limited resources were disadvantaged most. Medicaid, for example, was designed to alleviate the burden of lack of access to care but in reality, the low-income patient still has other challenges to overcome to access care. Roe v. Wade brought to light the challenges women have when access to safe abortions is limited. This is not just a US problem but globally, where women with low resources are more likely to be hospitalized or even worse die from complications of an unsafe abortion. Finally, we have all learned about issues that originate from policies that are implemented based on resources available to the majority in the US Precious time elapsed getting the vaccine to low income, disabled, and computer illiterate persons because of a policy that was implemented for the majority of persons known to have computers, cars, and access to public transportation.

Chapter Review Questions

1. *Which of the following social determinants from the Four-Pillar SDOH Framework (Social, Cultural, Environment, Policy) is most relevant to Mrs. James situation?*

    Mrs. James is a 54-year-old African American breast cancer survivor who described being especially vulnerable to contracting this virus which could prove deadly given her immunocompromised system. Mr. James spoke of the stress from not being able to adhere to the physical distancing guidelines from living with other family members who were not as careful with adhering to COVID-19 guidelines. Adhering to guidelines while living in a household with family members who were frontline workers or in occupations where social distancing was a challenge was especially frightening for these women. Mrs. James spoke of the threat of contracting COVID-19 from her family:

    Because you know it's up in the air. This virus is so unknown that you know we don't know what the effects are for people who have our own immune-suppressed medications and not only that my age and all this kind of stuff so I'm very stressed out. I have not been out of the house more than twice in 2 or 3 weeks. And when I do go out I wear my mask or gloves and stuff. And I'm not even in contact with anybody that has gone out. I don't even do a lot of contact with my husband. My children. None of that. Because you know I just want to isolate myself. Because I don't want to be exposed. And that in itself not getting out, not going around doing stuff that's stressful in itself.

2. *Which of the following social determinants from the Four-Pillar SDOH Framework (Social, Cultural, Environment, Policy) is most relevant to Mr. Langston's situation?*

    Mr. Langston was an 88-year-old African American who grew up during segregation in the Southern USA. He recalled ways in which white residents discouraged African Americans from continuing their education beyond what was necessary for employment in jobs that required the skill set for working as a domestic or laborer. Reportedly, while white employers were encouraging their descendants and white employees to attend college, they would communicate to their African American employees that there was no need for a college education. Both Mr. Langston and his Dad were workers on a farm and were paid very low wages for long hours of hard physical labor. Mr. Langston overheard a conversation between his Dad and the employer detailing why the young interviewee did not need a college education.

    I grew up during segregation and there was only one Black high school. The county furnished buses for the white kids, but if we Black kids wanted to go to high school, we had to walk 4 miles one way. After high school, I thought about going to college but the white man my father worked for talked my father out of it. Meanwhile, the white man's son went to Clemson.

Answers

1. *Environment and Policy*: Mrs. James is aware of the CDC Guidelines for physical distancing but not able to adhere to those guidelines since she has no control over who is living in her home. The CDC guidelines do not consider that individuals may live in a household with other family members and not able to adhere to physical distancing guidelines.
2. *Social and Policy*: The Jim Crow Laws enforced in the Southern US supported racial segregation in public institutions. The result of these racist laws prevented African Americans from obtaining a quality education or even from being able to attend college. Even though Jim Crow ended in 1968, those racist policies have had a lasting effect on inequities in education.

References

1. World Health Organization. Social determinants of health. 2022. https://www.who.int/health-topics/social-determinants-of-health#tab=tab_1. Accessed 29 Sept 2022.
2. Solar O, Irwin A. A conceptual framework for action on the social determinants of health. Social determinants of health discussion paper 2 (policy and practice). Discussion paper series on social determinants of health. August 29, 2022 ed. Geneva: World Health Organization; 2010.
3. Mangold KA, Bartell TR, Doobay-Persaud AA, Adler MD, Sheehan KM. Expert consensus on inclusion of the social determinants of health in undergraduate medical education curricula. Acad Med. 2019;94:1355–60.
4. Mangold KA, Williams AL, Ngongo W, et al. Expert consensus guidelines for assessing students on the social determinants of health. Teach Learn Med. 2022:1–9.
5. Doobay-Persaud A, Adler MD, Bartell TR, et al. A community of practice for teaching the social determinants of health in undergraduate medical education. J Gen Intern Med. 2020;35:1315–6.
6. Doobay-Persaud A, Adler MD, Bartell TR, et al. Teaching the social determinants of health in undergraduate medical education: a scoping review. J Gen Intern Med. 2019;34:720–30.
7. U. S. Department of Health and Human Services, Office of Disease Prevention and Health Promotion. Social determinants of health. https://health.gov/healthypeople/objectives-and-data/social-determinants-health. Accessed 29 Aug 2022.
8. Scarneo-Miller SE, DiStefano LJ, Singe SM, Register-Mihalik JK, Stearns RL, Casa DJ. Emergency action plans in secondary schools: barriers, facilitators, and social determinants affecting implementation. J Athl Train. 2020;55:80–7.
9. Nguyen KH, Cemballi AG, Fields JD, Brown W, Pantell MS, Lyles CR. Applying a socio-ecological framework to chronic disease management: implications for social informatics interventions in safety-net healthcare settings. JAMIA Open. 2022;5:ooac014.
10. Choi J, Park J, Kim JE, et al. Socioecological approach for identifying the determinants of objectively measured physical activity: a prospective study of the UK Biobank. Prev Med. 2022;155:106949.
11. NIMHD research framework 2017. https://nimhd.nih.gov/researchFramework. Accessed 29 Aug 2022.
12. U.S. Department of Health & Human Services. Racism and health. 2021. https://www.cdc.gov/healthequity/racism-disparities/index.html. Accessed 6 Sept 2022.

13. Rouse JA. Lugenia burns hope: Black southern reformer. Athens, GA: The University of Georgia Press; 1989.
14. The Atlantic. America's health segregation problem: has the country done enough to overcome its Jim Crow health care system? 2016. https://www.theatlantic.com/politics/archive/2016/05/americas-health-segregation-problem/483219/
15. Gamble VN. Germs have no color line: Blacks and American medicine, 1900–1940. New York: Garland Publishing, Inc.; 1989.
16. Byrd WM, Clayton LA. Race, medicine, and health care in the United States: a historical survey. J Natl Med Assoc. 2001;93:11S–34S.
17. Jones J. Labor of love, labor of sorrow. New York: Vintage Books; 1995.
18. Giddings P. When and where I enter: the impact of Black women on race and sex in America. New York: William Morrow; 1984.
19. Lovett BL. America's Historically Black Colleges & Universities: a narrative history, 1837–2009. Macon, GA: Mercer University Press; 2015.
20. Hamilton JB. Black Appalachia's oldest: untold stories of racism, religion and mental health. 2022.
21. Gerend MA, Pai M. Social determinants of Black-White disparities in breast cancer mortality: a review. Cancer Epidemiol Biomark Prev. 2008;17:2913–23.
22. Bhambhvani HP, Peterson DJ, Sheth KR. Sociodemographic factors associated with Wilms tumor treatment and survival: a population-based study. Int Urol Nephrol. 2022;54(12):3055–62.
23. Moubadder L, Collin LJ, Nash R, et al. Drivers of racial, regional, and socioeconomic disparities in late-stage breast cancer mortality. Cancer. 2022;128:3370–82.
24. Tran R, Forman R, Mossialos E, Nasir K, Kulkarni A. Social determinants of disparities in mortality outcomes in congenital heart disease: a systematic review and meta-analysis. Front Cardiovasc Med. 2022;9:829902.
25. Yadav RS, Chaudhary D, Avula V, et al. Social determinants of stroke hospitalization and mortality in United States' counties. J Clin Med. 2022;11:4101.
26. Jemal A, Thun MJ, Ward EE, Henley SJ, Cokkinides VE, Murray TE. Mortality from leading causes by education and race in the United States, 2001. Am J Prev Med. 2008;34:1–8.
27. Walsemann KM, Bell BA. Integrated schools, segregated curriculum: effects of within-school segregation on adolescent health behaviors and educational aspirations. Am J Public Health. 2010;100:1687–95.
28. Lincoln AK, Eyllon M, Prener C, et al. Prevalence and predictors of limited literacy in public mental health care. Community Ment Health J. 2021;57:1175–86.
29. Ajuwon AM, Insel K. Health literacy, illness perception, depression, and self-management among African Americans with type 2 diabetes. J Am Assoc Nurse Pract. 2022;34:1066–74.
30. Thomson MD, Williams AR, Sutton AL, Tossas KY, Garrett C, Sheppard VB. Engaging rural communities in cancer prevention and control research: development and preliminary insights from a community-based research registry. Cancer Med. 2021;10:7726–34.
31. Largent EA. Public health, racism, and the lasting impact of hospital segregation. Public Health Rep. 2018;133:715–20.
32. Gillispie-Bell V. The contrast of color: why the Black community continues to suffer health disparities. Obstet Gynecol. 2021;137:220–4.
33. Kaufman HW, Niles JK, Nash DB. Disparities in SARS-CoV-2 positivity rates: associations with race and ethnicity. Popul Health Manag. 2020;24(1):20–6.
34. Hamilton JB, Stewart BJ, Crandell JL, Lynn MR. Development of the ways of helping questionnaire: a measure of preferred coping strategies for older African American cancer survivors. Res Nurs Health. 2009;32:243–59.
35. Hermence B. Before freedom: 48 oral histories of former North and South Carolina slaves. Winston-Salem, NC: John F. Blair; 1990.
36. Powdermaker H. After freedom: a cultural study in the deep south. Madison, WS: University of Wisconsin Press; 1937.

37. Hamilton JB, Sandelowski M. Types of social support among African American cancer patients. Oncol Nurs Forum. 2004;31:792–800.
38. Poussaint AF, Alexander A. Lay my burden down: unraveling suicide and the mental health crisis among African Americans. Boston, MA: Beacon Press Books; 2000.
39. Carlton-LaNey I, Hamilton J, Ruiz D, Alexander S. Sitting with the sick: African American women's philanthropy. Affilia. 2001;16:447–66.
40. Haas KB. Forgotten veterinarians, 4. John Boyd Dunlop and his pneumatic tire. Vet Herit. 2005;28:10–2.
41. Hamilton JB, Worthy VC, Moore AD, Best NC, Stewart JM, Song MK. Messages of hope: helping family members to overcome fears and fatalistic attitudes toward cancer. J Cancer Educ. 2015;32(1):190–7.
42. Disparities in wealth by race and ethnicity in the 2019 survey of consumer finances. Washington, DC: Board of Governors of the Federal Reserve System; 2020. https://www.federalreserve.gov/econres/notes/feds-notes/disparities-in-wealth-by-race-and-ethnicity-in-the-2019-survey-of-consumer-finances-20200928.html. Accessed 16 Sept 2022.
43. American Cancer Society. Cancer facts & figures for African Americans 2019–2021. Atlanta: American Cancer Society; 2019.
44. Alcala HE. Differential mental health impact of cancer across racial/ethnic groups: findings from a population-based study in California. BMC Public Health. 2014;14:930.
45. Sklenarova H, Krumpelmann A, Haun MW, et al. When do we need to care about the caregiver? Supportive care needs, anxiety, and depression among informal caregivers of patients with cancer and cancer survivors. Cancer. 2015;121:1513–9.
46. Schoenfeld ER, Francis LE. Word on the street: engaging local leaders in a dialogue about prostate cancer among African Americans. Am J Mens Health. 2015;10(5):377–88.
47. Rositch AF, Atnafou R, Krakow M, D'Souza G. A community-based qualitative assessment of knowledge, barriers, and promoters of communicating about family cancer history among African-Americans. Health Commun. 2018;34:1–10.
48. Traeger L, Cannon S, Keating NL, et al. Race by sex differences in depression symptoms and psychosocial service use among non-Hispanic Black and White patients with lung cancer. J Clin Oncol. 2014;32:107–13.
49. Somayaji D, Cloyes KG. Cancer fear and fatalism: how African American participants construct the role of research subject in relation to clinical cancer research. Cancer Nurs. 2015;38:133–44.
50. Pew Forum. On views of race and inequality, Black and Whites are worlds apart 2016 June 27. 2016.
51. Blair IV, Havranek EP, Price DW, et al. Assessment of biases against Latinos and African Americans among primary care providers and community members. Am J Public Health. 2013;103:92–8.
52. Moore AD, Hamilton JB, Knafl GJ, et al. Patient Satisfaction Influenced by interpersonal treatment and communication for African American men: the North Carolina-Louisiana Prostate Cancer Project (PCaP). Am J Mens Health. 2012;6:409–19.
53. Moore AD, Hamilton JB, Knafl GJ, et al. The influence of mistrust, racism, religious participation, and access to care on patient satisfaction for African American men: the North Carolina-Louisiana Prostate Cancer Project. J Natl Med Assoc. 2013;105:59–68.
54. Koenig HG, King DE, Carson VB. Handbook of religion and health. New York: Oxford University Press; 2012.
55. Idler E, Blevins J, Kiser M, Hogue C. Religion, a social determinant of mortality? A 10-year follow-up of the Health and Retirement Study. PLoS One. 2017;12:e0189134.
56. Reed PG. An emerging paradigm for the investigation of spirituality in nursing. Res Nurs Health. 1992;15:349–57.
57. Britt KC, Kwak J, Acton G, Richards KC, Hamilton J, Radhakrishnan K. Measures of religion and spirituality in dementia: an integrative review. Alzheimers Dement (NY). 2022;8:e12352.
58. Pew Forum. A religious portrait of African-Americans. Pew Forum on religion & public life. 2007.

59. Raboteau AJ. A fire in the bones: reflections on African-American religious history. Boston, MA: Beacon Press; 1995.

60. Miller TN, Matthie N, Best NC, Price MA, Hamilton JB. Intergenerational influences on faith-based strategies used in response to racial discrimination among young African American adults. J Natl Med Assoc. 2020;112:176–85.

61. Hamilton JB, Fluker WE. An exploration of suffering and spirituality among older African American cancer patients as guided by Howard Thurman's theological perspective on spirituality. J Relig Health. 2021;60(4):2810–29.

62. Chung B, Meldrum M, Jones F, Brown A, Jones L. Perceived sources of stress and resilience in men in an African American community. Prog Community Health Partnersh. 2014;8:441–51.

63. Teti M, Martin AE, Ranade R, et al. "I'm a keep rising. I'm a keep going forward, regardless": exploring Black men's resilience amid sociostructural challenges and stressors. Qual Health Res. 2012;22:524–33.

64. Raboteau AJ. Slave religion. The "invisible institution" in the Antebellum South. New York: Oxford University Press; 1978.

65. Walker WT. Somebody's calling my name. Black sacred music and social change. Valley Forge, PA: Judson Press; 1979.

66. Cone JH. The spirituals and the blues. Maryknoll, NY: Orbis Books; 2008.

67. Pinn AB. Why lord? Suffering and evil in Black theology. New York: Continuum; 1999.

68. Reagon BJ. If you don't go don't hinder me. The African American sacred song tradition. University of Nebraska Press: Bison Books; 2001.

69. Hamilton JB, Galbraith KV, Best NC, Worthy VC, Moore LT. African-American cancer survivors' use of religious beliefs to positively influence the utilization of cancer care. J Relig Health. 2015;54:1856–69.

70. Lambe CE. Complementary and alternative therapy use in breast cancer: notable findings. J Christ Nurs. 2013;30:218–25.

71. Sterba KR, Burris JL, Heiney SP, Ruppel MB, Ford ME, Zapka J. "We both just trusted and leaned on the Lord": a qualitative study of religiousness and spirituality among African American breast cancer survivors and their caregivers. Qual Life Res. 2014;23(7):1909–20.

72. Henderson P, Gore SV, Davis BL, Condon EH. African American women coping with breast cancer: a qualitative analysis. Oncol Nurs Forum. 2003;30:641–7.

73. Hamilton J, Powe B, Pollard A, Lee K, Felton A. Spirituality among African American cancer survivors. Cancer Nurs. 2007;30:309–16.

74. Maliski SL, Connor SE, Williams L, Litwin MS. Faith among low-income, African American/ Black men treated for prostate cancer. Cancer Nurs. 2010;33:470–8.

75. DiIorio C, Steenland K, Goodman M, Butler S, Liff J, Roberts P. Differences in treatment-based beliefs and coping between African American and white men with prostate cancer. J Community Health. 2011;36:505–12.

76. Colón-López V, Valencia-Torres IM, Ríos EI, Llavona J, Vélez-Álamo C, Fernández ME. Knowledge, attitudes, and beliefs about colorectal cancer screening in Puerto Rico. J Cancer Educ. 2022; https://doi.org/10.1007/s13187-022-02153-z.

77. Guariglia L, Ieraci S, Villani V, et al. Coping style in glioma patients and their caregiver: evaluation during disease trajectory. Front Neurol. 2021;12:709132.

78. Bengtson VL, Copen CE, Putney NM, Silverstein M. A longitudinal study of the intergenerational transmission of religion. Int Sociol. 2009;24 https://doi.org/10.1177/02685809091029.

79. American Cancer Society. Cancer facts and figures. Atlanta, GA. 2019.

80. Hamilton JB, Best NC, Galbraith KV, Worthy VC, Moore LA. Strategies African-American cancer survivors use to overcome fears and fatalistic attitudes. J Cancer Educ. 2014;30(4):629–35.

81. Degazon CE. Ethnic identification, social support and coping strategies among three groups of ethnic African elders. J Cult Divers. 1994;1:79–85.

82. Tessaro I, Eng E, Smith J. Breast cancer screening in older African-American women: qualitative research findings. Am J Health Promot. 1994;8:286–92.

83. Abdullah T, Brown TL. Mental illness stigma and ethnocultural beliefs, values, and norms: an integrative review. Clin Psychol Rev. 2011;31:934–48.
84. Haynes TF, Cheney AM, Sullivan JG, et al. Addressing mental health needs: perspectives of African Americans living in the rural south. Psychiatr Serv. 2017;68:573–8.
85. Columbia University Department of Psychiatry. Addressing mental health in the Black Community. 2019. https://www.columbiapsychiatry.org/news/addressing-mental-health-black-community. Accessed 1 Oct 2022.
86. USC School of Social Work. Why mental health care is stigmatized in Black Communities. 2019. https://dworakpeck.usc.edu/news/why-mental-health-care-stigmatized-black-communities. Accessed 1 Oct 2022.
87. Gary FA. Stigma: barrier to mental health care among ethnic minorities. Issues Ment Health Nurs. 2005;26:979–99.
88. Conner KO, Lee B, Mayers V, et al. Attitudes and beliefs about mental health among African American older adults suffering from depression. J Aging Stud. 2010;24:266–77.
89. Rivera KJ, Zhang JY, Mohr DC, Wescott AB, Pederson AB. A narrative review of mental illness stigma reduction interventions among African Americans in The United States. J Ment Health Clin Psychol. 2021;5:20–31.
90. Taylor RJ, Chatters L, Woodward AT, Boddie S, Peterson GL. African Americans' and Black Caribbeans' religious coping for psychiatric disorders. Soc Work Public Health. 2021;36:68–83.
91. McCauley L, Hayes R. From Florence to fossil fuels: nursing has always been about environmental health. Nurs Outlook. 2021;69:720–31.
92. Greenberg M. Hurricane Katrina: a signature cascading risk event and a warning. Am J Public Health. 2020;110:1493–4.
93. EPA. Climate change indicators: weather and climate. https://www.epa.gov/climate-indicators/weather-climate. Accessed 21 Sept 2022.
94. Giudice LC, Llamas-Clark EF, DeNicola N, et al. Climate change, women's health, and the role of obstetricians and gynecologists in leadership. Int J Gynaecol Obstet. 2021;155:345–56.
95. Du J, Cui L, Ma Y, et al. Extreme cold weather and circulatory diseases of older adults: a time-stratified case-crossover study in Jinan. China Environ Res. 2022;214:114073.
96. Kim KN, Lim YH, Bae S, et al. Associations between cold spells and hospital admission and mortality due to diabetes: a nationwide multi-region time-series study in Korea. Sci Total Environ. 2022;838:156464.
97. Zhou Y, Pan J, Xu R, et al. Asthma mortality attributable to ambient temperatures: a case-crossover study in China. Environ Res. 2022;214:114116.
98. Berberian AG, Gonzalez DJX, Cushing LJ. Racial disparities in climate change-related health effects in the United States. Curr Environ Health Rep. 2022;9:451–64.
99. Clougherty JE, Burris HH. Rising global temperatures is likely to exacerbate persistent disparities in preterm birth. Paediatr Perinat Epidemiol. 2022;36:23–5.
100. Yoo EH, Eum Y, Gao Q, Chen K. Effect of extreme temperatures on daily emergency room visits for mental disorders. Environ Sci Pollut Res Int. 2021;28:39243–56.
101. Fisher JA, Jiang C, Soneja SI, Mitchell C, Puett RC, Sapkota A. Summertime extreme heat events and increased risk of acute myocardial infarction hospitalizations. J Expo Sci Environ Epidemiol. 2017;27:276–80.
102. Environmental Protection Agency. Chemicals and toxics topics. 2022. https://www.epa.gov/environmental-topics/chemicals-and-toxics-topics. Accessed 23 Sept 2022.
103. Allgood KL, Mack JA, Novak NL, Abdou CM, Fleischer NL, Needham BL. Vicarious structural racism and infant health disparities in Michigan: the Flint Water Crisis. Front Public Health. 2022;10:954896.
104. Roy S, Edwards MA. Are there excess fetal deaths attributable to waterborne lead exposure during the Flint Water Crisis? Evidence from bio-kinetic model predictions and Vital Records. J Expo Sci Environ Epidemiol. 2022;32:17–26.

105. Reuben A, Moreland A, Abdalla SM, et al. Prevalence of depression and posttraumatic stress disorder in Flint, Michigan, 5 years after the onset of the water crisis. JAMA Netw Open. 2022;5:e2232556.

106. Bohnert AM, Nicholson LM, Mertz L, Bates CR, Gerstein DE. Green schoolyard renovations in low-income urban neighborhoods: benefits to students, schools, and the surrounding community. Am J Community Psychol. 2022;69:463–73.

107. Putra I, Astell-Burt T, Feng X. Association between built environments and weight status: evidence from longitudinal data of 9589 Australian children. Int J Obes. 2022;46:1534–43.

108. Gu X, Keller J, Zhang T, et al. Disparity in built environment and its impacts on youths' physical activity behaviors during COVID-19 pandemic restrictions. J Racial Ethn Health Disparities. 2022:1–11.

109. Child ST, Kaczynski AT, Fair ML, et al. 'We need a safe, walkable way to connect our sisters and brothers': a qualitative study of opportunities and challenges for neighborhood-based physical activity among residents of low-income African-American communities. Ethn Health. 2019;24:353–64.

110. Brookings. Unequal opportunity: race and education. 1998. https://www.brookings.edu/articles/unequal-opportunity-race-and-education/. Accessed 18 Sept 2022.

111. The persistence of racial segregation. 2021. https://www.facinghistory.org/educator-resources/current-events/persistence-racial-segregation-american-schools

112. Economic Policy Institute. Schools are still segregated, and black children are paying a price. 2020. https://www.epi.org/publication/schools-are-still-segregated-and-black-children-are-paying-a-price/. Accessed 18 Sept 2022.

113. Jackson H, Engelman M. Deaths, disparities, and cumulative (dis)advantage: how social inequities produce an impairment paradox in later life. J Gerontol A Biol Sci Med Sci. 2022;77:392–401.

114. The George Washington University. New study finds severe lack of diversity in the health care workforce. 2021. https://gwtoday.gwu.edu/new-study-finds-severe-lack-diversity-health-care-workforce

115. Hynson E, Bloomer J, Samson Z, Price K, Tran D, Muench U. Workforce trends of underrepresented minority nurses in the United States over the last decade: progress towards equal representation? Policy Polit Nurs Pract. 2022;23(4):215–27. https://doi.org/10.1177/15271544221118319.

116. The Century Foundation. Racism, inequality, and health care for African Americans. 2019. https://tcf.org/content/report/racism-inequality-health-care-african-americans/?session=1. Accessed 16 Sept 2022.

117. CDC. COVID-19 cases, hospitalization, and death by race/ethnicity. Atlanta, GA. 2020.

118. Sonik RA, Herrera AL. Associations between inspections for unsafe housing conditions and evictions in New York City public housing buildings(). J Community Health. 2022;47:849–52.

119. Chu MT, Fenelon A, Rodriguez J, Zota AR, Adamkiewicz G. Development of a multidimensional housing and environmental quality index (HEQI): application to the American Housing Survey. Environ Health. 2022;21:56.

120. Frazer E, Mitchell RA Jr, Nesbitt LS, et al. The violence epidemic in the African American community: a call by the National Medical Association for comprehensive reform. J Natl Med Assoc. 2018;110:4–15.

121. Blassingame JW. The slave community. Plantation life in the ante-bellum south. New York: Oxford University Press; 1972.

122. Lincoln CE, Mamiya LH. The Black Church in the African American experience. Durham, NC: Duke University Press; 1995.

123. Boles JB. Black Southerners, 1619–1869. Lexington, KY: The University Press of Kentucky; 1984.

124. Billingsley A. Black families in white America. New Jersey: Prentice-Hall; 1968.

125. Hill RB. The strengths of African-American families: twenty-five years later. Baltimore, MD: R & B Publishers; 1997.

126. McAdoo HP, Crawford V. The Black Church and family support programs. Prev Hum Serv. 1991;9:193–203.

127. Leone LA, Allicock M, Pignone MP, et al. Cluster randomized trial of a church-based peer counselor and tailored newsletter intervention to promote colorectal cancer screening and physical activity among older African Americans. Health Educ Behav. 2016;43:568–76.

128. Maxwell AE, Lucas-Wright A, Santifer RE, Vargas C, Gatson J, Chang LC. Promoting cancer screening in partnership with health ministries in 9 African American churches in South Los Angeles: an implementation pilot study. Prev Chronic Dis. 2019;16:E128.

129. Barg FK, Gullatte MM. Cancer support groups: meeting the needs of African Americans with cancer. Semin Oncol Nurs. 2001;17:171–8.

130. Chatters LM, Taylor RJ, Woodward AT, Nicklett EJ. Social support from church and family members and depressive symptoms among older African Americans. Am J Geriatr Psychiatry. 2015;23:559–67.

131. Corley AMS, Gomes SM, Crosby LE, et al. Partnering with faith-based organizations to offer flu vaccination and other preventive services. Pediatrics. 2022;150:e2022056193.

132. Knott CL, Chen C, Bowie JV, et al. Cluster-randomized trial comparing organizationally tailored versus standard approach for integrating an evidence-based cancer control intervention into African American churches. Transl Behav Med. 2022;12:673–82.

133. Moore D, Mansfield LN, Onsomu EO, Caviness-Ashe N. The role of black pastors in disseminating COVID-19 vaccination information to Black communities in South Carolina. Int J Environ Res Public Health. 2022;19:8926.

134. Nwaozuru U, Obiezu-Umeh C, Diallo H, et al. Perceptions of COVID-19 self-testing and recommendations for implementation and scale-up among Black/African Americans: implications for the COVID-19 STEP project. BMC Public Health. 2022;22:1220.

135. Rogers CR, Rogers TN, Matthews P, et al. Psychosocial determinants of colorectal cancer screening uptake among African-American men: understanding the role of masculine role norms, medical mistrust, and normative support. Ethn Health. 2022;27:1103–22.

136. Brewer LC, Jenkins S, Hayes SN, et al. Community-based, cluster-randomized pilot trial of a cardiovascular mobile health intervention: preliminary findings of the FAITH! Trial. Circulation. 2022;146:175–90.

137. Azibo D. Understanding the proper and improper usage of the comparative research framework. In: Burlew AKH, Banks WC, McAdoo HP, Azibo D, editors. African American psychology: theory, research, and practice. Newbury Park, CA: Sage; 1992. p. 5–27.

138. Dilworth-Anderson P. Extended kin networks in Black families. Generations. 1992;16:29–32.

139. Pew Research Center. On views of race and inequality, Blacks and Whites are worlds apart. 2016. https://www.pewresearch.org/social-trends/2016/06/27/1-demographic-trends-and-economic-well-being/. Accessed 19 Sept 2022.

140. Morton P. Disfigured images. Westport, CT: Praeger Publishers; 1991.

141. Taylor RJ, Chatters LM, Jackson JS. Changes over time in support network involvement among Black Americans. In: Taylor RJ, Chatters LM, Jackson JS, editors. Family life in Black America. Thousand Oaks, CA: Sage; 1997. p. 295–318.

142. A & E Television Networks, LLC. "Jim Crow Laws". History. 2022. https://www.history.com/topics/early-20thcentury-us/jim-crow-laws.

143. Gates J, Louis H. Stony the road: reconstruction, white supremacy, and the rise of Jim Crow. New York: Penguin Press; 2019.

144. Brown L, Valk A. Living with Jim Crow: African American women and memories of the segregated south. New York: Palgrave Macmillan; 2010.

145. Woodward CV. The strange life of Jim Crow. New York: Oxford University Press; 2002.

146. Hswen Y, Qin Q, Williams DR, Viswanath K, Brownstein JS, Subramanian SV. The relationship between Jim Crow laws and social capital from 1997–2014: a 3-level multilevel hierarchical analysis across time, county and state. Soc Sci Med. 2020;262:113142.

147. Smedley BD, Stith AY, Colburn L, Evans CH, Institute of Medicine (US). The right thing to do, the smart thing to do: enhancing diversity in the health professions: summary of the symposium on diversity in Health Professions in Honor of Herbert W Nickens, MD. Washington,

DC: National Academies Press (US); 2001. Copyright 2001 by the National Academy of Sciences. All rights reserved.

148. Hua CL, Bardo AR, Brown JS. Mistrust in physicians does not explain Black-White disparities in primary care and emergency department utilization: the importance of socialization during the Jim Crow era. J Natl Med Assoc. 2018;110:540–6.

149. Kaufman JC. The health consequences of Black subordination and White domination: a relational and located approach to studying the health of US older adults born 1938–1948. Dissertation. 2021.

150. Desegregation: the hidden legacy of Medicare. US News & World Report. 2015. https://www.usnews.com/news/articles/2015/07/30/desegregation-the-hidden-legacy-of-medicare. Accessed 1 Oct 2022.

151. The US Department of Health and Human Services (HHS). In: HHS, editor. Medicare and Medicaid. Washington, DC: HHS; 2022.

152. The US Department of Health and Human Services (HHS). Health insurance reform. Washington, DC: HHS; 2022.

153. Kim G, Qin J, Hall CB, In H. Association between socioeconomic and insurance status and delayed diagnosis of gastrointestinal cancers. J Surg Res. 2022;279:170–86.

154. Zaveri S, Nevid D, Ru M, et al. Racial disparities in time to treatment persist in the setting of a comprehensive breast center. Ann Surg Oncol. 2022;29:6692–703.

155. Stankowski TJ, Schumacher JR, Hanlon BM, et al. Barriers to breast reconstruction for socioeconomically disadvantaged women. Breast Cancer Res Treat. 2022;195:413–9.

156. Patel CG, Williams SP, Tao G. Access to healthcare and the utilization of sexually transmitted infections among homeless Medicaid patients 15 to 44 years of age. J Community Health. 2022;47:853–61.

157. Encyclopaedia Britannica. Roe v. Wade. 2022. https://www.britannica.com/event/Roe-v-Wade. Accessed 1 Oct 2022.

158. Cameron S. Recent advances in improving the effectiveness and reducing the complications of abortion. F1000Res. 2018;7:F1000.

159. Grimes DA, Benson J, Singh S, et al. Unsafe abortion: the preventable pandemic. Lancet. 2006;368:1908–19.

160. Rasch V. Unsafe abortion and postabortion care—an overview. Acta Obstet Gynecol Scand. 2011;90:692–700.

161. World Health Organization. Abortion. 2021. https://www.who.int/news-room/fact-sheets/detail/abortion. Accessed 27 Sept 2022.

162. Clarke D, Mühlrad H. Abortion laws and women's health. J Health Econ. 2021;76:102413.

163. Centers for Disease Control. Basics of COVID-19. 2021. https://www.cdc.gov/coronavirus/2019-ncov/your-health/about-covid-19/basics-covid-19.html#:~:text=COVID%2D19%20(coronavirus%20disease%202019,%2C%20a%20flu%2C%20or%20pneumonia. Accessed 27 Sept 2022.

164. World Health Organization. WHO coronavirus (COVID-19) dashboard. 2022. https://covid19.who.int/. Accessed 27 Sept 2022.

165. Maness SB, Merrell L, Thompson EL, Griner SB, Kline N, Wheldon C. Social determinants of health and health disparities: COVID-19 exposures and mortality among African American people in the United States. Public Health Rep. 2021;136:18–22.

166. Reyes VM. The disproportional impact of COVID-19 on African Americans. Health Hum Rights. 2020;22:299–307.

167. Centers for Disease Control and Prevention. COVID-19 vaccine equity. 2022. https://www.cdc.gov/coronavirus/2019-ncov/community/health-equity/vaccine-equity.html. Accessed 27 Sept 2022.

168. Moore JX, Gilbert KL, Lively KL, et al. Correlates of COVID-19 vaccine hesitancy among a community sample of African Americans living in the Southern United States. Vaccines (Basel). 2021;9:879.

169. Willis DE, Andersen JA, Bryant-Moore K, et al. COVID-19 vaccine hesitancy: race/ethnicity, trust, and fear. Clin Transl Sci. 2021;14:2200–7.

170. Balasuriya L, Santilli A, Morone J, et al. COVID-19 vaccine acceptance and access among Black and Latinx Communities. JAMA Netw Open. 2021;4:e2128575.
171. Reverby SM. Racism, disease, and vaccine refusal: people of color are dying for access to COVID-19 vaccines. PLoS Biol. 2021;19:e3001167.
172. Njoku A, Joseph M, Felix R. Changing the narrative: structural barriers and racial and ethnic inequities in COVID-19 vaccination. Int J Environ Res Public Health. 2021;18:9904.
173. United States Census Bureau. Computer and internet use in the United States: 2018. 2021. https://www.census.gov/newsroom/press-releases/2021/computer-internet-use.html. Accessed Press Release Number CB21-TPS.38, 2022.
174. American Public Transportation Association. Public transportation facts. 2022. https://www.apta.com/news-publications/public-transportation-facts/. Accessed 29 Sept 2022.
175. Economic Policy Institute. Who are essential workers? A comprehensive look at their wages, demographics, and unionization rates. 2020. https://www.epi.org/blog/who-are-essential-workers-a-comprehensive-look-at-their-wages-demographics-and-unionization-rates/. Accessed 29 Sept 2022.

Canvas Faculty Development Site

3

Adarsh Char

Learning Objectives

- Explain the course design approach used to develop the faculty professional development SDOH course.
- Connect the rationale behind how the SDOH course was built to faculty members' own course development efforts.
- Reflect on how to introduce SDOH into nursing curriculum in an LMS context.
- Identify the impact of offering faculty a resource to develop and include SDOH topics in their own courses.

Introduction

The consideration of Social Determinants of Health (SDOH) in Nursing Education is an obvious and important addition to the already brimful curriculum that both undergraduate and graduate nursing students must undertake. No matter their path forward in the field of nursing; be it practice, research, leadership, or teaching, nursing students must be able to evaluate and act on the cultural, social, environmental, and public policy contexts, as articulated elsewhere in this text, which can and do affect health outcomes.

While we know that we want future nurses to have a clear sense of the fact that health equity gaps can affect health outcomes, beyond that surface awareness, how do we determine that they will use that awareness to apply a broader lens to their practice; that they will widen the aperture on their research observations; that they will make better, data-driven decisions for the patients their organizations care for;

A. Char (✉)
Full Tilt Ahead, Arlington, VA, USA

Nell Hodgson Woodruff School of Nursing, Emory University, Atlanta, GA, USA
e-mail: achar2@emory.edu

© The Author(s), under exclusive license to Springer Nature Switzerland AG 2023
J. B. Hamilton et al. (eds.), *Integrating a Social Determinants of Health Framework into Nursing Education*, https://doi.org/10.1007/978-3-031-21347-2_3

or that they will continue teaching diversity, equity, and inclusion? This central question of how to make actionable the awareness of SDOH is the foundation on which we built this course for faculty.

Application of the SDOH and the four pillars is the key aim of this course. We want faculty to be able to apply the SDOH lens to their own courses and, by extension, operationalize the consideration of SDOH into the learning their students are doing. Specifically, we want students to be able to evaluate and determine if and how SDOH were considered in the learning materials such as texts, articles, case studies, research studies, and data, that they encounter. In addition, we want students to be able to use that SDOH lens when completing course assessments, i.e., use an SDOH lens when responding to discussion questions, completing an essay, redesigning an intake form, developing a presentation, or taking a test. The goal then, is to leave our students with a practiced approach to thinking more broadly about the way that they practice nursing.

In this course, faculty are guided on how to modify the assignments and assessments in their own courses to consider an SDOH lens. For example, a patient case study presentation that required a student to develop a case that helps illustrate how a patient may present with a topic condition could be modified slightly to also consider the specific populations most affected by the condition and also note health disparities that might cause an increased prevalence of such a condition. In this way, faculty can assess students' understanding of SDOH and its impacts. This also illustrates that the work required of faculty is not an onerous one—the idea is not to rebuild their courses from the ground up, but rather to scaffold their existing teaching so that their students' consideration of social determinants of health is a thread woven through the courses they teach now.

As Barak Rosenshine, emeritus professor of education psychology at the University of Illinois, noted in his 2010 report for UNESCO, *Principles of Instruction*, "The most successful teachers spent more time in guided practice, more time asking questions, more time checking for understanding, and more time correcting errors" [1]. This is poignant because this is precisely what our faculty do with their students now, and what we determined to be the best way to enhance what our faculty know about SDOH and how to implement it in their own courses. Following the first introduction to SDOH and the Four Pillars, we invited faculty to post an assignment or activity idea that they think addresses one of the Four Pillars and then subsequently respond to their colleagues' posts about assignments and activity ideas they had posted.

The course also invited faculty to build a community of practice around SDOH by sharing not only assignment ideas but also articles, research, and other academic resources that address or consider SDOH. While we encouraged them to build a library of such resources that were specific to their areas of specialty, we also included many of the resources they brought forward in the Handbook that was distributed to all faculty at the conclusion of the course.

Incorporating SDOH as part of the nursing curriculum at Emory Nursing may have been undertaken in many ways. But the most effective approach was multipronged. The direct guidance from the School's leadership, a critically important factor for the success of this effort, launched simultaneous action across various parts of the organization. The first step included the Curriculum Committee introducing the SDOH goal into every syllabus for every course offered at the school. In addition, time and resources were allocated to develop the SDOH course that all faculty were required to complete. While the course was being developed, Dr. Hamilton, who developed the Four Pillars framework, was also invited to give lectures on the framework for groups of students and faculty. Finally, a subsequent result of the course is a Handbook that is available to all faculty offering an indexed reference for every type of assignment, i.e., essay, discussion, presentation, and case study, and which SDOH pillar(s) it addresses.

Course Design

The SDOH course for faculty was designed as a 3-part course in Emory Nursing Professional Development Center's Canvas Learning Management System. The course includes three modules: an Introduction to Social Determinants of Health, a module on Addressing Instruction, and a module on Considering Learning.

We introduce faculty to the course with specific goals we want to meet by the end of the course. These include:

- Knowing what Social Determinants of Health (SDOH) are in a global context.
- Being able to differentiate between the universal context of Social Determinants of Health and the Four Pillars we focus on at Emory Nursing.
- Being able to recognize and transition student activities, assignments, and assessments to consider an SDOH lens.
- Being able to help their students identify and evaluate data, research, articles, and other instructional artifacts for consideration of SDOH.
- Valuing and helping their students value the need to identify and mitigate health care disparities across populations.

We also introduce faculty to this course with a strong recommendation to partner with any number of other faculty members who will be engaging with this course. This will help support their learning and provide effective peer review of their assignment and resource recommendations. In addition, we ask faculty to grow this partnership into a community of practice across the School that can continue to improve learning materials and sources shared with students and highlight effective approaches they may have undertaken in their courses to incorporate SDOH.

Part 1: Introduction to Social Determinants of Health—Pre-test

The first module includes a low-stakes, ungraded, pre-test that asks faculty to consider what they know already about SDOH. As an example, one question asks: "A faculty member is developing a lecture focused on pandemics and wants to incorporate the 4 pillars of SDOH into their lecture. The lecture focuses on the influences from the social conditions that explain racial disparities in outcomes from COVID-19. Which influences might the faculty member consider? Select all that apply." Possible choices include Income, Education, Access to health care, and Religion. Questions such as these served to gauge what faculty already knew about SDOH as well as to allow them to make some predictive inferences about what they were going to learn in this course.

Other questions asked faculty why they thought it was important to incorporate SDOH into the curriculum. While this is not fundamental to incorporating SDOH into their curriculum, it is important in understanding motivation. While the majority of faculty selected the right reasons such as helping to address pervasive inequities in health care and the necessity of meeting the needs of diverse population in practice, some also believed that this was necessary for accreditation or that it was a part of the University's mission. Maehr, M. and Meyer, H. (1997) note that "Motivation is the personal investment an individual is willing to make to reach some desired state or outcome" [2]. That motivation is what influences what learners pay attention to or focus on, directs their attention to the task at hand and prevents distractions, helps them persist, and helps them monitor their own learning [3]. So, understanding what our faculty's motivations are helped guide how SDOH was introduced to them and how we focused on operationalizing the task at hand, i.e., weaving SDOH into their current teaching practice.

Part 1: Introduction to Social Determinants of Health—Interactive Learning

The primary course content was built using an industry-standard tool known and Articulate Rise which offers interactive learning components such as hotspot images, tabs, sliders, and other ways to chunk information into more manageable pieces (See Fig. 3.1).

This first module is segmented into two lessons: The first introduces Social Determinants of Health in a global context, including references to other sources that have defined SDOH such as Artiga and Hinton [4], the US Department of Health and Human Services' Healthy People 2030 report, the Centers for Disease Control and Prevention, and the WHO. In this segment, we also cover why SDOH are important and why the American Association of Colleges of Nursing (AACN) believes nurses must have a more nuanced understanding of the complex and less obvious drivers of health.

SOCIAL	ENVIRONMENTAL	CULTURAL	POLICY

Social Conditions can be defined as those that occur in society due to systemic racism, economic disparities, education gaps, and/or occupations that influence wellness. Specifically, we consider:

- Access to education, finacial resources, job opportunities
- Social Support
- Language and Health literacy
- Access to health care (use of preventive health services, primary care)
- Incarceration

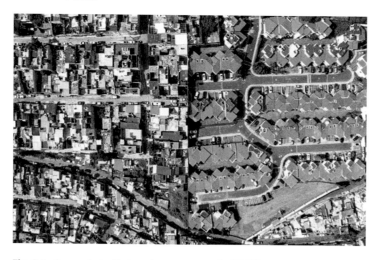

Fig. 3.1 Screenshot of interactive component in SDOH course for faculty

The second lesson dives deeper into the Four Pillars framework developed by Dr. Jill B. Hamilton. In this lesson, faculty are offered more detailed views into how the various components of SDOH were reorganized and simplified to develop a useful and pragmatic framework to guide nursing education. In particular, a key learning point illustrates the high-priority health topics that correspond to pediatric, young adult/adult, and older adult/geriatric patients.

Part 2: Addressing Instruction—Interactive Learning

We begin Part 2 of the course with an interactive lesson that is a practical guide to implementation. The lesson dives into providing faculty with instructional activities that are aligned with the Four Pillars. As they navigate through the specific assignments and activities we highlight, they are asked to consider how the assignments and activities they present to their students might be modified to consider a view through the SDOH lens.

The lesson invites faculty to explore activities such as discussing race in the classroom and assigning anti-racism reading and writing reflections to address the Social Conditions pillar. Under the Environmental Conditions pillar, we invite faculty to ensure more clinical rotations in settings where SDOH are often assessed and addressed simultaneously with clinical care provision or to provide opportunities to shadow case management or social work to understand the work, scope, and resources of allied-health professionals who address SDOH.

To promote the Cultural Conditions pillar, faculty are asked to try to provide and/ or encourage more community/cultural immersion nursing clinical rotation activities. And the Policy Conditions pillar recommends direct involvement in government through attendance and reflection on local, state, and federal public meetings that discuss health policy impacting SDOH. Faculty are also introduced to other learning activities that address one or more of the SDOH framework pillars such as modifying intake/screening forms, nursing diagnoses and care plan recommendations, and developing a library of community-specific resources that can be made available to patients.

The learning content for Part 2 concludes with specific example assignments for faculty to explore that are accompanied by a detailed explanation of the assignment, a rationale, alignment to AACN Essentials and necessary resources or links to resources that students may need to use in order to complete the assignment. This exploration of assignments such as the field observations assignment, conflict outcome journals, care plan recommendations, and pathophysiological evaluation provided a rich field of the types of assignments and activities that faculty would discussion in their first community of practice assignment.

Part 2: Addressing Instruction—Incorporating SDOH into Teaching Practice Discussion

The second component of Part 2 of the SDOH course for faculty included a discussion with peers about incorporating SDOH into their teaching practice. In the lesson they just completed, we had faculty explore specific examples of SDOH in their teaching practice and consider assignment examples and activities that will prompt students to apply an SDOH lens to their work.

In this discussion assignment, we asked faculty to post an assignment or activity idea that they think addresses one of the Four Pillars. Faculty were then prompted to respond to their colleague's posts about their assignment or activity idea.

We invited faculty to upload an assignment on which they would like peer feedback. We also reminded them to work in groups to complete this exercise and go through a round of peer feedback before moving on to the next module in this course.

The discussion assignment, then, was more than just an opportunity to discuss how-to strategies but rather an opportunity to practice what they would be doing across each of their courses and get near-immediate feedback. As noted previously, a key goal of this course is to help faculty be able to recognize and transition student activities, assignments, and assessments to consider an SDOH lens. This assignment provided that practice.

The results were significant. All faculty participants responded to the discussion with assignments or activity examples. A key benefit of this was the free exchange of ideas and feedback provided not only by Dr. Hamilton and others who are studied in this topic, but also by peers who nudged, guided, corrected, or influenced each other with their recommendations and suggestions in replies. In addition, many provided resources, texts, articles, and other sources that could be used to introduce SDOH into existing curriculum.

Part 3: Considering Learning—Interactive Learning

Critical consciousness, as initially proposed by Brazilian educator and author of Pedagogy of the Oppressed, Paulo Freire, suggests a process by which individuals become aware of societal inequities and as a result, take action to dismantle those structures and systems that promote them [5]. In their 2018 article, Sharma et al. suggest a refocus on critical consciousness in medical education. By recentering the conversation about SDOH around justice and inequity, they suggest that we can "deepen collective understanding of power, privilege, and the inequities embedded in social justice among medical trainees." In other words, rather than incremental shifts in a curriculum that introduce race but not racism, or transgender studies but not transphobia, or poverty but not oppression, that a major structural and cultural transformation needs to take place in medical education in order for organizations to become truly socially responsible [6].

In Part 3 of our course, we fine-tune the lens for faculty. In the previous module, we introduced how to migrate the faculty's own teaching practice to include a more conspicuous consideration of Social Determinants of Health. In this module, we look more toward our students' practice of learning. How do they know when an article considers SDOH? Are certain resources better than others in identifying gaps in health outcomes across populations? Can students pick out for themselves how the authors of studies, research, and papers structured their work to include more than just a surface-level nod to social determinants of health?

This module, then, looks to evaluate the "critical consciousness" that Sharma describes by providing exemplars of the sorts of readings that students should look at more deeply in order to understand how to identify the consideration of SDOH and to determine if that consideration is a mere a nod in the direction of health inequities or if it represents a structural and cultural transformation.

The module begins with example articles and readings that are categorized into the Four Pillars. For each reading, we identify the population or setting on which the article focuses. In addition, we identify the specific social determinant addressed in the article, and the findings. For example, see Tables 3.1 and 3.2.

Table 3.1 Example article addressing SDOH

Naegle, M. A., et al., 2020. Opioid crisis through the lens of social justice
Population/setting: Problems exemplified among impoverished populations, rural, and underserved
Social determinant: Social Pillar. Disparities in access to health care services, preventive care
Findings: Safe pain management, social justice in resources in pain management and substance abuse treatment. The widespread obstacles to equitable access to multimodal pain management and comprehensive, evidence-based treatment and support services for vulnerable populations with OUDs and at-risk populations are in conflict with the principles of social justice. These obstacles include limited access to care, failure to recognize the full scope of practice for APRNs, inadequate funding streams, inadequate comprehensive health professional education on pain and the risks associated with opioid use and widespread public, professional, and political stigma experienced by these vulnerable populations [7]

Table 3.2 Example article addressing SDOH

Duque, RB, 2020. *Black Health Matters Too… Especially in the Era of Covid-19: How Poverty and Race Converge to Reduce Access to Quality Housing, Safe Neighborhoods, and Health and Wellness Services and Increase the Risk of Co-morbidities Associated with Global Pandemics*
Population/setting: Minority populations in community settings in Utica, New York
Social determinant: Environmental Pillar. Poor neighborhoods/intergenerational influences on poverty
Findings: Analysis of data related to overlapping obstacles like lack of access to safe housing and quality health services offers both context and insight into how policies addressing poverty reduction may offer pathways for reducing the co-morbidities associated with pandemic risk for African Americans [8]

Part 3: Considering Learning—Building a Community of Practice Discussion

The aim of providing these readings by SDOH pillar is to help faculty connect the dots between what an article is about and where it might fit into their existing curriculum. As with the modifications of assignments, a reflection on one of the articles noted above versus another that simply merely outlines a picture of the findings on pain management or health access is an easy modification that can have a tremendous impact on students' awareness of health disparities.

After having just reviewed SDOH-related resources that faculty can introduce into their courses we ask them to share some of their own resources. Whereas in the previous lesson we looked at how to assign work to students that prompted them to consider SDOH, in this lesson, we consider the kinds of resources to which we can introduce our students that make the addressing of SDOH common practice.

We do this through another community of practice discussion where we ask faculty to post a link to an article, research paper, dataset, or other academic resources that address or consider SDOH. In particular, we ask them to consider resources that not only point out disparities or health inequities but also offer mitigation strategies. We then prompt them to respond to one of their colleague's posts about their resource. A key point of this discussion is to begin building a library of resources with their colleagues that might be useful in their collective teaching practice. As with the previous discussion addressing assignments and articles, this one resulted in a broad and deep collection of resources.

As an example, one faculty member, Dr. Ann-Marie Brown pointed out, "One of the challenges I have identified is finding pictorial representation of a variety of backgrounds and skin tones when preparing a PP or other kind of presentation for students (or a conference, etc.). A particular issue is making sure we look at what various skin lesions look like across many skin tones and types. This article is a great help—Maymone MBC, Watchmaker JD, Dubiel M, Wirya SA, Shen LY & Vashi NA. 2019. Common skin disorders in pediatric skin of color. Journal of Pediatric Health Care, Vol 33, Issue 6, pgs 727–737. It addresses the disparities in presentation and thus recognition, but also treatment."

The Community of Practice discussion resulted in hundreds of resources being offered along with each faculty's expertly considered rationale for why the resource was important and what aspects of SDOH it addressed. In isolation, each of these resources may have been used by the instructor and perhaps others who we introduced to it in a one-on-one setting. But the introduction of these resources through this course aided rapid dissemination across all faculty in two ways: Not only did it spur conversation and analysis in the discussion itself to provide additional context and consideration, but it also made it possible for us to develop the Handbook which includes citations of these resources for long-term use.

Post-test and Handbook

The final components of this course include a post-test administered to all faculty as a measure of course completion and a resulting Handbook that was produced after the course was concluded.

While the results of the post-test were significant, we will not delve too deeply into the results here. It is important to note, however, that the key indicator of success for the team that developed and implemented the course was that the mean score moved from 61 to 84% overall. In addition, an analysis of each of the items on the test showed that participants moved from the 60–79% quintile to the 80–100% quintile. This is important because of the ten questions presented on the test, eight were multiple answer questions, i.e., select all that apply, and only two were multiple choice questions. This indicated that not only were faculty more knowledgeable about the SDOH and Four Pillars, but that their knowledge is more nuanced because their mean earned scores on individual multiple answer questions improved from the range of 0.36–0.78 out of 1 point to a range 0.70–0.97 points out of 1 on each question.

The accompanying handbook (included as an appendix to this text) is a compilation of assignment and lecture ideas that were shared by Emory School of Nursing faculty and students who participated in the SDOH course along with other curated assignment ideas.

The assignments in the handbook were compiled and organized by assignment type and by the SDOH Pillar(s) that they address. Each assignment includes the pillars supported by that assignment, information about the assignment, and any objectives that may have been included in the assignment.

Assignment types include:

- Interactive: Assignments that are hands-on, experiential, or completed through simulation and/or group activities.
- Personal reflection: Assignments that require students to reflect on personal thoughts, perspectives, or feelings.
- Research: Assignments that require students to look up, analyze, and synthesize information.
- Writing: Assignments that have a writing component.
- Open discussion: Assignments that have a component where students can share their thoughts, findings, or perspectives in a group forum.
- Reading: Assignments that have required reading (books, articles, etc.).
- Lecture: Shared during or as part of a classroom lecture.
- Presentation: Assignment that requires a student to develop and share presentations.

In addition, the Handbook also includes Resources. Resources are the SDOH-related articles, data, websites, research, etc. that would be valuable for students to engage with in considering SDOH topics.

Summary

Using a backward integrated design, we were able to identify the key aims of the SDOH course, determine the assessments that we would use to help faculty and the administration at Emory Nursing know that faculty had met those goals, and then develop the course materials that would be presented.

All faculty at the School were required to complete the course and the administrative mandate made the course a success in terms of:

- Educating faculty on SDOH.
- Introducing them to the Four Pillars that we focus on at Emory Nursing.
- Helping faculty understand and practice how to modify their own course assignments and assessments to incorporate an SDOH lens in order to ensure that students have a deeper understanding of the causes of health disparities and the structural changes that are necessary to mitigate them.
- Helping faculty identify and teach their own students how to identify resources that consider SDOH.
- Helping to spread the consideration of SDOH in their students' future nursing practice.

The result of this initiative is a comprehensive approach to curricular change—from in-person lectures, to this interactive course, to the ready reference, faculty and students should find it much easier to be able to practice critical consciousness and help promote positive health outcomes to the diverse populations they serve.

Authors' Contributions   Adarsh Char designed and developed the SDOH course for faculty and students. Dr. Jill B. Hamilton provided the source instructional content, Dr. Autherine Abiri and Priya Schaffner gathered and compiled assignment examples and resources used in the course.

Appendix

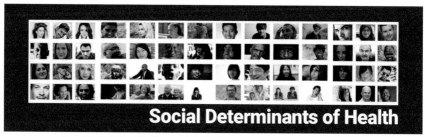

Emory Nursing's Four Pillar Framework for Teaching and Learning about Social Determinants of Health

Assignments for Course Integration

Developed by
Dr. Jill B. Hamilton
Adarsh Char
Dr. Wanjira Kinuthia
Dr. Autherine Abiri
Priya Schaffner

E = Environmental	S = Social
C = Cultural	P = Policy

Table of Contents

Contents

Table of Contents 2
About this handbook 5
How to use this manual 5
How to cite this resource 5
The Four Pillars Explained 6
    Social 6
    Environmental 6
    Cultural 7
    Policy 7
Assignments by Pillar 8
    Environmental 8
    Social 9
    Cultural 11
    Policy 12
Assignments by Type 14
    Interactive 14
    Personal reflection 14
    Research 14
    Writing 15
    Open discussion 16
    Reading 17
    Lecture 17
    Presentation 17
    Resource 17
Assignment Details 19
    Assignment: Immersive Learning Experience 19
    Assignment: Bill Identification and Introduction 19
    Assignment: Journal Article Critique 20
    Assignment: Addressing Social Determinants of Health in Pharmacology 20
    Assignment: Understanding How Public Schools/Programs are Funded 21
    Assignment: Adapting Health History Tool 21
    Assignment: Addressing SDOH in SOAPIE Notes 21

E = Environmental	S = Social
C = Cultural	P = Policy

Assignment: SDOH Pediatric Case Study and Presentation 22

Assignment: Understanding Disparities in Accessing Pain Management 23

Assignment: Impact of SDOH on Validating Classification and Risk Models... 23

Assignment: An Examination of Environmental Justice 24

Assignment: Mapping Inequality Redlining in New Deal 24

Assignment: Mitigating Impact of Bullying on Mental Health on LGBTQ Youth.. 24

Assignment: Incorporating SDOHs into Clinical Interview 25

Assignment: Social Determinants of Health-Based Critique of Measures Used in Research 25

Assignment: Incorporating SDOH Into Lectures and Assignments... 26

Assignment: Addressing SDOHs in Complex Case Studies 26

Assignment: Addressing Racism in Pediatric Practice 27

Assignment: Incorporating SDOH Assessment into Windshield Survey 27

Assignment: Culturally-Sensitive Risk and Protective Factors for Mental Health 28

Assignment: Addressing SDOHs in SOAP Note.. 28

Assignment: Understanding Impact of Environmental/Policy Determinants on Patient's Health 28

Assignment: Access to Resources by Zip Code... 29

Assignment: Clinically Competent and Culturally Proficient Care for Transgender and Gender
Nonconforming Patients... 29

Assignment: Shadowing a Social Worker 30

Assignment: Sharing Our Stories 30

Assignment: Health Disparities and Maternal Morbidity... 30

Assignment: Exploring Racial Disparities in Women's Health Care Group Presentation.............................. 32

Assignment: Foot Care for the Homeless 32

Assignment: PREPARE Tool for SDOH Assessment 33

Assignment: SDOH Planning During Patient Discharge 33

Assignment: Understanding Connection Between Food Insecurity and Obesity 33

Assignment: Health Advocacy Assignment 34

Assignment: Nursing Values in Micro-System Assessment 35

Assignment: SDOH Assessment in Ambulatory Care Setting.. 35

Assignment: How Geography Impacts Access 35

Assignment: Brainstorming Research Topics That Address SDOH of Patient Population............................ 36

Assignment: Holistic Patient Planning Case Study.. 36

Assignment: Addressing SDOH in Midwifery Case Study 36

Assignment: Reflecting on how SDOH Impact Mental Health Outcomes 37

Assignment: SDOH Influences on the Rate and Causes of Maternal Mortality 38

Assignment: Impact of SDOH on Health Outcomes of Adult Patients and Veterans 38

E = Environmental	S = Social
C = Cultural	P = Policy

Assignment: Patient Case Study and Presentation 38
Assignment: Trauma Informed Care Discussion 39
Assignment: Advocating to Policy Makers 39
Assignment: Capturing SDOHs in Emory EMR 39
Assignment: Assessing Racial and Ethnic Disparities in Obstetric Anesthesia 40
Assignment The Role of SDOH in Symptom Management 40
Assignment: SOAP Note with SDOH Planning 40
Assignment: How SDOH Impact maternal mortality in Georgia 40
Assignment: SDOH Planning for Surgical Patients 41
Assignment: The Accountable Health Communities Health-Related Social Needs Screening Tool............ 41
Assignment: Reading and Reflection: Monique and the Mango Rains... 41
Assignment: Racial and/or Ethnic Disparities in Pregnancy 42
Assignment: SDOH Impact on the LGBTQIA+ Population 42
Assignment: Understanding How Health Equity is Addressed in Epidemiological Concepts 43
Assignment: Discussing SDOH as Part of Pediatric Simulation 43
Assignment: How SDOH Contribute to Health Disparities 44
Assignment: Ambulatory Clinical Debrief 45
Assignment: Developing Theoretical Framework with SDOH Components 46
Assignment: Economic Inequality Map 46
Assignment: Addressing SDOH in DNP Project Proposal 46
Assignment: Systems Thinking Approach to address SDOH.. 48
Assignment: Ethical Practice in Research Design 48
Assignment: Care Plan Assignment.. 48
Assignment: Impact of SDOH in Data Analysis... 49
Assignment: Adding SDOH Pillars to Ambulatory Intake Form 49
Assignment: Development of a Centering Pregnancy Module on Maternal Mortality: Focus on
Cardiovascular Conditions During Pregnancy 50
Assignment: Using SDOH Lens to Choose Research Questions 51
Assignment: Live Simulation on Health Equity... 51
Assignment: Social and Cultural Considerations in Advance Directive Planning............................ 51
Assignment: Examining Social and Environmental Factors That Impact Sleep 51
Assignment: Medical/Surgical Rotation SDOH Assessment 52
Assignment: SOAP Note: Integrating SDOH Into Planning 52

E = Environmental	S = Social
C = Cultural	P = Policy

About this handbook

The **Social Determinants of Health** (SDOH) course was developed in 2021 by **Dr. Jill Hamilton, Adarsh Char, Dr. Autherine Abiri, Dr. Wanjira Kinuthia,** and **Priya Schaffner** to offer Emory School of Nursing faculty and students an application-based approach to incorporating Emory Nursing's Four Pillar Framework for teaching and learning about social determinants of health.

The authors would like to thank the faculty at the Nell Hodgson Woodruff School of Nursing for their participation and contributions to this project.

This manual is a compilation of assignment and lecture ideas that were shared by Emory School of Nursing faculty and students who participated in the SDOH course along with other curated assignment ideas.

The assignments in this handbook have been compiled and organized by **assignment type** and by the **SDOH Pillar(s)** that they address. Each assignment includes the pillars supported by that assignment, information about the assignment, and any objectives that may have been included for the assignment.

Assignment types include:
- **Interactive**: Assignments that are hands-on, experiential, or completed through simulation and/or group activities
- **Personal reflection**: Assignments that require students to reflect on personal thoughts, perspectives, or feelings
- **Research**: Assignments that require students to look-up, analyze, and synthesize information
- **Writing**: Assignments that have a writing component
- **Open discussion**: Assignments that have a component where students can share their thoughts, findings, or perspectives in a group forum
- **Reading**: Assignments that have required reading (books, articles, etc.)
- **Lecture**: Shared during or as part of a class-room lecture
- **Presentation**: Assignment that requires student to develop and share presentations

In addition, we have also included **Resources**. Resources are not assignments but rather some SDOH-related resource that would be valuable for students to engage with.

How to use this manual

There are two tables of content below. The first shows all the assignments in this handbook organized by **SDOH pillar**. The other is organized by **assignment type**. Each table of contents lists the assignments that correspond with the various categories and these assignments can be accessed by clicking the hyperlink from the table of contents.

How to cite this resource

Hamilton, J. B., Char, Adarsh S., Kinuthia, W., Abiri, A., Schaffner, P. (2022). Handbook of Assignments for SDOH Course Integration. Nell Hodgson Woodruff School of Nursing.

E = Environmental	S = Social
C = Cultural	P = Policy

The Four Pillars Explained

The four pillars identified in the Emory Nursing SDOH Framework are a synthesis of several widely recognized SDOH frameworks from organizations and scholars in this field such as S. Artiga and E. Hinton (2018), the Centers for Disease Control and Prevention, the US Department of Health and Human Services, and the World Health Organization.

While the frameworks developed by these organizations address many of the conditions that are determinants of health, such as environmental conditions, socio-economic conditions, racism and diversity, etc., they do not individually cover the broad spectrum of conditions that impact health outcomes.

The Emory Nursing SDOH Framework reorganizes and simplifies the key areas of social determinants to offer a useful and pragmatic framework to guide nursing education as follows:

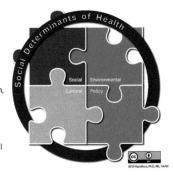

Social

Social Conditions can be defined as those that occur in society due to systemic racism, economic disparities, education gaps, and/or occupations that influence wellness. Specifically, we consider:

- Access to education, financial resources, job opportunities
- Social Support
- Language and Health literacy
- Access to health care (use of preventive health services, primary care)
- Incarceration

Environmental

Physical environments have an outsized impact on individual and population health. In the Emory Nursing SDOH Framework, we consider the following:
- Natural environment: Green space, buildings, bike lanes, sidewalks, lighting, trees, benches
- Exposure to toxic substances
- Access to foods that support healthy eating patterns
- Natural resources: Climate, weather, air pollution
- Naturally occurring social interactions/social connections
- Familial relationships
- Social capital

Here, we also consider the social environment (social settings) in which people live that influence wellness:
- Faith-based institutions
- Health care settings

E = Environmental	S = Social
C = Cultural	P = Policy

- Quality of schools, academic settings
- Worksites, schools, recreational settings
- Housing (safe and quality housing), community design (physical barriers)
- Crime and violence
- Access to affordable transportation
- Recreational resources--Safe play spaces

Cultural

Customary beliefs, social norms, attitudes, values, practices shared by a group of people (community or society) in a place and time can affect health outcomes. In particular, cultural conditions that can influence SDOH include:

- Religion/spirituality
- Societal values
- Nursing values
- Interpersonal Racism/Discrimination
- Customs/behaviors
- Identity (ethnicity, gender, sexual orientation)

Policy

Guidelines, principles, legislation and activities that affect the living conditions conducive to the welfare of individuals', communities', and societies' quality of life make up the Fourth Pillar of the Emory Nursing SDOH Framework: Policy. This pillar considers the policies that affect social issues such as:

- Affordable/universal health insurance
- Child protection
- Abortion
- Guns
- Sex workers
- LGBTQ issues (including same sex marriage)
- Education/housing policies
- Recreational drugs
- APRN restrictions (e.g., restriction on prescriptions, radiology, dispensing, collaborating physician)

E = Environmental	S = Social
C = Cultural	P = Policy

Assignments by Pillar

Environmental

- Immersive Learning Experience
- Journal Article Critique
- Addressing Social Determinants of Health in Pharmacology
- Understanding How Public Schools/Programs are Funded
- Adapting Health History Tool
- Addressing SDOH in SOAPIE Notes
- SDOH Pediatric Case Study and Presentation
- Understanding Disparities in Accessing Pain Management
- Impact of SDOH on Validating Classification and Risk Models
- An Examination of Environmental Justice
- Mapping Inequality Redlining in New Deal
- Incorporating SDOHs into Clinical Interview
- Social Determinants of Health-Based Critique of Measures Used in Research
- Incorporating SDOH Into Lectures and Assignments
- Addressing SDOHs in Complex Case Studies
- Incorporating SDOH Assessment into Windshield Survey
- Culturally Sensitive Risk and Protective Factors for Mental Health
- Addressing SDOHs in SOAP Note
- Understanding Impact of Environmental/Policy Determinants on Patient's Health
- Access to Resources by Zip Code
- Shadowing a Social Worker
- Health Disparities and Maternal Morbidity
- Exploring Racial Disparities in Women's Health Care Group Presentation
- Foot Care for the Homeless
- PREPARE Tool for SDOH Assessment
- SDOH Planning During Patient Discharge
- Understanding Connection Between Food Insecurity and Obesity
- SDOH Assessment in Ambulatory Care Setting
- How Geography Impacts Access
- Brainstorming Research Topics That Address SDOH of Patient Population
- Holistic Patient Planning Case Study
- Addressing SDOH in Midwifery Case Study
- Reflecting on how SDOH Impact Mental Health Outcomes
- SDOH Influences on the Rate and Causes of Maternal Mortality
- Impact of SDOH on health outcomes of adult patients and Veterans
- Patient Case Study and Presentation
- Capturing SDOHs in Emory EMR
- The Role of SDOH in Symptom Management
- SOAP Note with SDOH Planning
- How SDOH Impact maternal mortality in Georgia
- SDOH Planning for Surgical Patients

E = Environmental	S = Social
C = Cultural	P = Policy

- The Accountable Health Communities Health-Related Social Needs Screening Tool
- Reading and Reflection: Monique and the Mango Rains
- SDOH Impact on the LGBTQIA+ Population
- Understanding How Health Equity is Addressed in Epidemiological Concepts
- How SDOH Contribute to Health Disparities
- Ambulatory Clinical Debrief
- Developing Theoretical Framework with SDOH Components
- Economic Inequality Map
- Addressing SDOH in DNP Project Proposal
- Systems Thinking Approach to Address SDOH
- Ethical Practice in Research Design
- Care Plan Assignment
- Impact of SDOH in Data Analysis
- Adding SDOH Pillars to Ambulator Intake Form
- Development of a Centering Pregnancy Module on Maternal Mortality: Focus on Cardiovascular Conditions During Pregnancy
- Using SDOH Lens To Choose Research Questions
- Live Simulation on Health Equity
- Examining Social and Environmental Factors That Impact Sleep
- Medical/Surgical Rotation: SDOH Assessment
- SOAP Note: Integrating SDOH Into Planning

Social

- Immersive Learning Experience
- Journal Article Critique
- Addressing Social Determinants of Health in Pharmacology
- Adapting Health History Tool
- Addressing SDOH in SOAPIE Notes
- SDOH Pediatric Case Study and Presentation
- Impact of SDOH on Validating Classification and Risk Models
- An Examination of Environmental Justice
- Mapping Inequality Redlining in New Deal
- Mitigating Impact of Bullying on Mental Health on LGBTQ Youth
- Incorporating SDOHs into Clinical Interview
- Social Determinants of Health-Based Critique of Measures Used in Research
- Incorporating SDOH Into Lectures and Assignments
- Addressing SDOHs in Complex Case Studies
- Addressing Racism in Pediatric Practice
- Incorporating SDOH Assessment into Windshield Survey
- Culturally Sensitive Risk and Protective Factors for Mental Health
- Addressing SDOHs in SOAP Note
- Access to Resources by Zip Code
- Clinically Competent and Culturally Proficient Care for Transgender and Gender Nonconforming Patients
- Shadowing a Social Worker

E = Environmental	S = Social
C = Cultural	P = Policy

- Health Disparities and Maternal Morbidity
- Exploring Racial Disparities in Women's Health Care Group Presentation
- Foot Care for the Homeless
- PREPARE Tool for SDOH Assessment
- SDOH Planning During Patient Discharge
- Understanding Connection Between Food Insecurity and Obesity
- Nursing Values in Micro-System Assessment
- SDOH Assessment in Ambulatory Care Setting
- How Geography Impacts Access
- Brainstorming Research Topics That Address SDOH of Patient Population
- Holistic Patient Planning Case Study
- Addressing SDOH in Midwifery Case Study
- Reflecting on how SDOH Impact Mental Health Outcomes
- SDOH Influences on the Rate and Causes of Maternal Mortality
- Impact of SDOH on health outcomes of adult patients and Veterans
- Patient Case Study and Presentation
- Trauma Informed Care Discussion
- Capturing SDOHs in Emory EMR
- The Role of SDOH in Symptom Management
- SOAP Note with SDOH Planning
- How SDOH Impact maternal mortality in Georgia
- SDOH Planning for Surgical Patients
- The Accountable Health Communities Health-Related Social Needs Screening Tool
- Reading and Reflection: Monique and the Mango Rains
- Racial and/or Ethnic Disparities in Pregnancy
- SDOH Impact on the LGBTQIA+ Population
- Understanding How Health Equity is Addressed in Epidemiological Concepts
- Discussing SDOH as Part of Pediatric Simulation
- How SDOH Contribute to Health Disparities
- Ambulatory Clinical Debrief
- Developing Theoretical Framework with SDOH Components
- Economic Inequality Map
- Addressing SDOH in DNP Project Proposal
- Systems Thinking Approach to Address SDOH
- Ethical Practice in Research Design
- Care Plan Assignment
- Impact of SDOH in Data Analysis
- Adding SDOH Pillars to Ambulator Intake Form
- Development of a Centering Pregnancy Module on Maternal Mortality: Focus on Cardiovascular Conditions During Pregnancy
- Using SDOH Lens to Choose Research Questions
- Live Simulation on Health Equity
- Social and Cultural Considerations in Advance Directive Planning
- Examining Social and Environmental Factors That Impact Sleep
- Medical/Surgical Rotation: SDOH Assessment
- SOAP Note: Integrating SDOH Into Planning

E = Environmental	S = Social
C = Cultural	P = Policy

Cultural

- Immersive Learning Experience
- Journal Article Critique
- Addressing Social Determinants of Health in Pharmacology
- Adapting Health History Tool
- Addressing SDOH in SOAPIE Notes
- SDOH Pediatric Case Study and Presentation
- Impact of SDOH on Validating Classification and Risk Models
- Mapping Inequality Redlining in New Deal
- Mitigating Impact of Bullying on Mental Health on LGBTQ Youth
- Incorporating SDOHs into Clinical Interview
- Social Determinants of Health-Based Critique of Measures Used in Research
- Incorporating SDOH Into Lectures and Assignments
- Addressing SDOHs in Complex Case Studies
- Incorporating SDOH Assessment into Windshield Survey
- Culturally Sensitive Risk and Protective Factors for Mental Health
- Addressing SDOHs in SOAP Note
- Shadowing a Social Worker
- Sharing Our Stories
- Health Disparities and Maternal Morbidity
- Exploring Racial Disparities in Women's Health Care Group Presentation
- Foot Care for the Homeless
- PREPARE Tool for SDOH Assessment
- SDOH Assessment in Ambulatory Care Setting
- Brainstorming Research Topics That Address SDOH of Patient Population
- Holistic Patient Planning Case Study
- Addressing SDOH in Midwifery Case Study
- Reflecting on how SDOH Impact Mental Health Outcomes
- SDOH Influences on the Rate and Causes of Maternal Mortality
- Impact of SDOH on health outcomes of adult patients and Veterans
- Patient Case Study and Presentation
- Capturing SDOHs in Emory EMR
- Assessing Racial and Ethnic Disparities in Obstetric Anesthesia
- The Role of SDOH in Symptom Management
- SOAP Note with SDOH Planning
- How SDOH Impact maternal mortality in Georgia
- SDOH Planning for Surgical Patients
- The Accountable Health Communities Health-Related Social Needs Screening Tool
- Reading and Reflection: Monique and the Mango Rains
- Racial and/or Ethnic Disparities in Pregnancy
- SDOH Impact on the LGBTQIA+ Population
- Understanding How Health Equity is Addressed in Epidemiological Concepts
- Discussing SDOH as Part of Pediatric Simulation
- How SDOH Contribute to Health Disparities
- Ambulatory Clinical Debrief

E = Environmental	S = Social
C = Cultural	P = Policy

- Developing Theoretical Framework with SDOH Components
- Addressing SDOH in DNP Project Proposal
- Systems Thinking Approach to Address SDOH
- Ethical Practice in Research Design
- Care Plan Assignment
- Impact of SDOH in Data Analysis
- Adding SDOH Pillars to Ambulator Intake Form
- Development of a Centering Pregnancy Module on Maternal Mortality: Focus on Cardiovascular Conditions During Pregnancy
- Using SDOH Lens to Choose Research Questions
- Live Simulation on Health Equity
- Social and Cultural Considerations in Advance Directive Planning
- Medical/Surgical Rotation: SDOH Assessment
- SOAP Note: Integrating SDOH Into Planning

Policy

- Immersive Learning Experience
- Journal Article Critique
- Bill Identification and Introduction
- Addressing Social Determinants of Health in Pharmacology
- Understanding How Public Schools/Programs are Funded
- SDOH Pediatric Case Study and Presentation
- Understanding Disparities in Accessing Pain Management
- An Examination of Environmental Justice
- Mapping Inequality Redlining in New Deal
- Social Determinants of Health-Based Critique of Measures Used in Research
- Incorporating SDOH Into Lectures and Assignments
- Addressing SDOHs in Complex Case Studies
- Incorporating SDOH Assessment into Windshield Survey
- Culturally Sensitive Risk and Protective Factors for Mental Health
- Understanding Impact of Environmental/Policy Determinants on Patient's Health
- Shadowing a Social Worker
- Health Disparities and Maternal Morbidity
- Exploring Racial Disparities in Women's Health Care Group Presentation
- Foot Care for the Homeless
- Health Advocacy Assignment
- SDOH Assessment in Ambulatory Care Setting
- Brainstorming Research Topics That Address SDOH of Patient Population
- Holistic Patient Planning Case Study
- Addressing SDOH in Midwifery Case Study
- Reflecting on how SDOH Impact Mental Health Outcomes
- SDOH Influences on the Rate and Causes of Maternal Mortality
- Impact of SDOH on Health Outcomes of Adult Patients and Veterans
- Patient Case Study and Presentation
- Advocating to Policy Makers

E = Environmental	S = Social
C = Cultural	P = Policy

- Capturing SDOHs in Emory EMR
- The Role of SDOH in Symptom Management
- How SDOH Impact maternal mortality in Georgia
- Reading and Reflection: Monique and the Mango Rains
- **SDOH Impact on the LGBTQIA+ Population**
- Understanding How Health Equity is Addressed in Epidemiological Concepts
- How SDOH Contribute to Health Disparities
- Ambulatory Clinical Debrief
- Developing Theoretical Framework with SDOH Components
- Addressing SDOH in DNP Project Proposal
- Systems Thinking Approach to Address SDOH
- Care Plan Assignment
- Impact of SDOH in Data Analysis
- Adding SDOH Pillars to Ambulator Intake Form
- Development of a Centering Pregnancy Module on Maternal Mortality: Focus on Cardiovascular Conditions During Pregnancy
- Using SDOH Lens to Choose Research Questions
- Live Simulation on Health Equity

E = Environmental	S = Social
C = Cultural	P = Policy

Assignments by Type

Interactive

- Understanding Disparities in Accessing Pain Management
- Immersive Learning Experience
- Incorporating SDOHs into Clinical Interview
- Incorporating SDOH Into Lectures and Assignments
- Addressing SDOHs in Complex Case Studies
- Shadowing a Social Worker
- Foot Care for the Homeless
- SDOH Assessment in Ambulatory Care Setting
- Discussing SDOH as Part of Pediatric Simulation
- Systems Thinking Approach to Address SDOH
- Development of a Centering Pregnancy Module on Maternal Mortality: Focus on Cardiovascular Conditions During Pregnancy
- Live Simulation on Health Equity
- Examining Social and Environmental Factors That Impact Sleep
- Medical/Surgical Rotation: SDOH Assessment

Personal reflection

- Immersive Learning Experience
- Shadowing a Social Worker
- Holistic Patient Planning Case Study
- Reflecting on how SDOH Impact Mental Health Outcomes
- Impact of SDOH on health outcomes of adult patients and Veterans
- SDOH Impact on the LGBTQIA+ Population
- Ambulatory Clinical Debrief
- Social and Cultural Considerations in Advance Directive Planning
- Medical/Surgical Rotation: SDOH Assessment

Research

- Bill Identification and Introduction
- Journal Article Critique
- Understanding How Public Schools/Programs are Funded
- Adapting Health History Tool
- Addressing SDOH in SOAPIE Notes
- SDOH Pediatric Case Study and Presentation
- Understanding Disparities in Accessing Pain Management
- An Examination of Environmental Justice
- Mapping Inequality Redlining in New Deal

E = Environmental	S = Social
C = Cultural	P = Policy

- Mitigating Impact of Bullying on Mental Health on LGBTQ Youth
- Social Determinants of Health-Based Critique of Measures Used in Research
- Incorporating SDOH Assessment into Windshield Survey
- Access to Resources by Zip Code
- Health Disparities and Maternal Morbidity
- Exploring Racial Disparities in Women's Health Care Group Presentation
- SDOH Planning During Patient Discharge
- Health Advocacy Assignment
- Nursing Values in Micro-System Assessment
- SDOH Assessment in Ambulatory Care Setting
- How Geography Impacts Access
- Advocating to Policy Makers
- Capturing SDOHs in Emory EMR
- Assessing Racial and Ethnic Disparities in Obstetric Anesthesia
- The Role of SDOH in Symptom Management
- How SDOH Impact maternal mortality in Georgia
- Racial and/or Ethnic Disparities in Pregnancy
- Understanding How Health Equity is Addressed in Epidemiological Concepts
- How SDOH Contribute to Health Disparities
- Economic Inequality Map
- Addressing SDOH in DNP Project Proposal
- Adding SDOH Pillars to Ambulator Intake Form
- Using SDOH Lens to Choose Research Questions
- Examining Social and Environmental Factors That Impact Sleep

Writing

- Bill Identification and Introduction
- Journal Article Critique
- Understanding How Public Schools/Programs are Funded
- Adapting Health History Tool
- Addressing SDOH in SOAPIE Notes
- SDOH Pediatric Case Study and Presentation
- Mitigating Impact of Bullying on Mental Health on LGBTQ Youth
- Incorporating SDOHs into Clinical Interview
- Social Determinants of Health-Based Critique of Measures Used in Research
- Incorporating SDOH Assessment into Windshield Survey
- Addressing SDOHs in SOAP Note
- Understanding Impact of Environmental/Policy Determinants on Patient's Health
- Access to Resources by Zip Code
- SDOH Planning During Patient Discharge
- Health Advocacy Assignment
- Nursing Values in Micro-System Assessment
- SDOH Assessment in Ambulatory Care Setting
- How Geography Impacts Access

E = Environmental	S = Social
C = Cultural	P = Policy

- Brainstorming Research Topics That Address SDOH of Patient Population
- Holistic Patient Planning Case Study
- Addressing SDOH in Midwifery Case Study
- Reflecting on how SDOH Impact Mental Health Outcomes
- Impact of SDOH on Health Outcomes of Adult Patients and Veterans
- Advocating to Policy Makers
- Assessing Racial and Ethnic Disparities in Obstetric Anesthesia
- SOAP Note with SDOH Planning
- How SDOH Impact maternal mortality in Georgia
- SDOH Planning for Surgical Patients
- Reading and Reflection: Monique and the Mango Rains
- SDOH Impact on the LGBTQIA+ Population
- Understanding How Health Equity is Addressed in Epidemiological Concepts
- How SDOH Contribute to Health Disparities
- Ambulatory Clinical Debrief
- Developing Theoretical Framework with SDOH Components
- Economic Inequality Map
- Addressing SDOH in DNP Project Proposal
- Ethical Practice in Research Design
- Care Plan Assignment
- Impact of SDOH in Data Analysis
- Adding SDOH Pillars to Ambulator Intake Form
- Development of a Centering Pregnancy Module on Maternal Mortality: Focus on Cardiovascular Conditions During Pregnancy
- Medical/Surgical Rotation: SDOH Assessment
- SOAP Note: Integrating SDOH Into Planning

Open discussion

- Addressing Social Determinants of Health in Pharmacology
- Impact of SDOH on Validating Classification and Risk Models
- Mapping Inequality Redlining in New Deal
- Incorporating SDOH Into Lectures and Assignments
- Addressing SDOHs in Complex Case Studies
- Addressing Racism in Pediatric Practice
- Culturally Sensitive Risk and Protective Factors for Mental Health
- Sharing Our Stories
- Exploring Racial Disparities in Women's Health Care Group Presentation
- Foot Care for the Homeless
- Understanding Connection Between Food Insecurity and Obesity
- SDOH Influences on the Rate and Causes of Maternal Mortality
- Patient Case Study and Presentation
- Trauma Informed Care Discussion
- The Role of SDOH in Symptom Management
- SDOH Planning for Surgical Patients

E = Environmental	S = Social
C = Cultural	P = Policy

- Discussing SDOH as Part of Pediatric Simulation
- Ambulatory Clinical Debrief
- Live Simulation on Health Equity
- Social and Cultural Considerations in Advance Directive Planning
- Medical/Surgical Rotation: SDOH Assessment

Reading

- Incorporating SDOH Into Lectures and Assignments
- Health Disparities and Maternal Morbidity
- Reading and Reflection: Monique and the Mango Rains
- Understanding How Health Equity is Addressed in Epidemiological Concepts
- Adding SDOH Pillars to Ambulator Intake Form
- Development of a Centering Pregnancy Module on Maternal Mortality: Focus on Cardiovascular Conditions During Pregnancy

Lecture

- SDOH Pediatric Case Study and Presentation
- Incorporating SDOH Into Lectures and Assignments
- Clinically Competent and Culturally Proficient Care for Transgender and Gender Nonconforming Patients
- Health Disparities and Maternal Morbidity
- PREPARE Tool for SDOH Assessment
- Understanding Connection Between Food Insecurity and Obesity
- The Accountable Health Communities Health-Related Social Needs Screening Tool
- SDOH Impact on the LGBTQIA+ Population

Presentation

- SDOH Pediatric Case Study and Presentation
- Sharing Our Stories
- Exploring Racial Disparities in Women's Health Care Group Presentation
- Patient Case Study and Presentation
- The Role of SDOH in Symptom Management
- Racial and/or Ethnic Disparities in Pregnancy
- How SDOH Contribute to Health Disparities
- Systems Thinking Approach to Address SDOH

Resource

E = Environmental	S = Social
C = Cultural	P = Policy

- Health Disparities and Maternal Morbidity
- PREPARE Tool for SDOH Assessment
- The Accountable Health Communities Health-Related Social Needs Screening Tool
- Addressing SDOH in DNP Project Proposal

E = Environmental	S = Social
C = Cultural	P = Policy

Assignment Details

Assignment: Immersive Learning Experience
By: Elaine Fisher

SDOH Pillars Addressed	E ● S ● C ● P
Assignment Type	Interactive, Personal reflection
Assignment Details	Environmental: Have students ride a public bus that passes through multiple areas in downtown Atlanta. Observe the neighborhoods/transitions between neighborhoods observing for stores, general environment, people and activities in the area. Cultural: What observations do you make regarding who gets on and off the bus? What biases do your observations carry? Do you think the time-of-day impacts what you observed? How would this impact your assessment? How might this impact care you would provide to an individual if there were an emergency on the bus?
Assignment Objectives	

Assignment: Bill Identification and Introduction
By: Beth Ann Swan

SDOH Pillars Addressed	P
Assignment Type	Research, Writing
Assignment Details	Choose a National or State bill currently in the legislature. The bill must be current and related to health or social policy. Submit a brief (less than 10 minutes) presentation of the bill using 3 to 5 slides. The presentation must provide the following information: • What search tool did you use to find the bill? • The number and title of the bill • Purpose of the bill in 3 to 5 sentences • The body in which it was introduced (State or Federal, House or Senate) • Who introduced the bill and how many cosponsors? • Where is the bill in the legislative process? Is it in a Committee? Waiting for a floor vote? Is it in appropriations? Waiting for a Governor or Presidential signature? • Why is the bill of interest to you? • What is the impact/influence on professional practice?
Assignment Objectives	• Student will use various Bill search resources • Student will identify a bill of interest that is currently active in the legislature

E = Environmental	S = Social
C = Cultural	P = Policy

Assignment: Journal Article Critique
By: Irene Yang

SDOH Pillars Addressed	E ● S ● C ● P
Assignment Type	Research, Writing
Assignment Details	Article Critique – Directions
	Use the format provided below for the article critique. The completed assignment should not exceed one page, single spaced.
	Purpose/Hypothesis:
	State the hypothesis of the article and the hypothesis to be tested using the – omic focused approach. Is it clearly stated?
	Methods:
	Identify the design used in the study.
	Identify the research protocol used and how the authors may or may not have addressed the stated hypothesis.
	What is the inclusion/exclusion criteria?
	How did the researchers ensure validity and reliability of the omic data presented?
	Analysis, Interpretation and Ethics:
	Does the data analysis appear appropriate?
	Are appropriate graphics/visualizations used to illustrate the results?
	Do the authors reach a conclusion that is fully supported by the data presented? If not, what do the data support?
	Are there any ethical concerns? If so, how might the ethical concerns have been addressed?
	How does this research study address one of social determinants of health (see Emory SON Four Pillars) and/or have an impact on health equity? OR How could this study have been designed to better address an SDOH or have an impact on health equity?
	Reflection:
	What were the limitations of this study?
	What other -omic focus areas might have been useful in this study to test the hypothesis?
	Would these other areas offer any additional fidelity?
Assignment Objectives	

Assignment: Addressing Social Determinants of Health in Pharmacology
By: Kenneth Mueller

SDOH Pillars Addressed	Primary: C
	Secondary: E ● S ● P

E = Environmental	S = Social
C = Cultural	P = Policy

Assignment Type	Open Discussion
Assignment Details	The primary topic targeted is systemic racism starting with a focus on Race Based Medicine. During our first weeks of class, students watch a Ted Talk, "The Problem with Race Based Medicine," and discuss the history of the medication BiDil(R). This medication creates a false assumption that race is a proxy for biological determinants of health and skips over SDOH. Other potential areas of discussion include; • Food deserts and their consequences on diseases like hypertension, dyslipidemia and diabetes • Pharmacy deserts and their consequences on access to medicine, vaccines (like COVID-19) and even health screenings • The history of drug clinical trials and exclusion of patients across the lifespan (women, geriatrics, pediatrics and vulnerable and underserved populations) and so many more.
Assignment Objectives	

Assignment: Understanding How Public Schools/Programs are Funded
By: Lisa Marie Wands

SDOH Pillars Addressed	E ● P
Assignment Type	Research, Writing
Assignment Details	Examine public school districts and research how they are funded. Inequalities in school funding is a core foundation for perpetuating systemic racism.
Assignment Objectives	

Assignment: Adapting Health History Tool
By: Kristy Kiel Martyn

SDOH Pillars Addressed	E ● S ● C
Assignment Type	Research, Writing
Assignment Details	Health Assessment assignment: Select a standard health history tool, review, and identify SDOH assessment items included and needed. For SDOH assessment items identified as needed, develop questions to add to standard tools.
Assignment Objectives	

Assignment: Addressing SDOH in SOAPIE Notes
By: Patti Landerfelt

E = Environmental	S = Social
C = Cultural	P = Policy

SDOH Pillars Addressed	E ● S ● C
Assignment Type	Research, Writing
Assignment Details	Utilize the pathophysiologic evaluation assignment to encourage students to apply an SDOH lens to their patient assessment skills. Encourage students to write a SOAPIE note based on the patient's presenting signs and symptoms, history and physical assessment, pertinent or abnormal lab work, and the way in which the lab work correlates with the differential diagnosis. Add social components to the scenario by mentioning the fact that the patient does not have access to transportation to and from the healthcare facility, they do not have financial resources to pay for transportation or food for the day, and they also have fears surrounding their health and healthcare providers in general.
Assignment Objectives	

Assignment: SDOH Pediatric Case Study and Presentation
By: Sharron Close

SDOH Pillars Addressed	E ● S ● C ● P
Assignment Type	Research, Writing, Presentation, Lecture
Assignment Details	Address SDOH in the primary care setting through the presentation of a complex teaching case to be peer-evaluated. Students collaborate in pairs to create a comprehensive teaching case that will be shared and peer-evaluated by the class. This assignment is designed to guide student immersion into consideration of social, environmental, cultural and policy implications during the course of real-life pediatric primary care practice. • Present a comprehensive complex teaching case that includes HPI, ROS, PE, Differential Considerations, Include Images or Labs, Final Diagnosis with ICD 10 code, Review of Illness or Disease, Treatment Plan supported by current guidelines or evidence. Give level of service code. • Choose a Social Determinant of Health and discuss how that SDOH* may impact the Past History, HPI, ROS, PE and treatment plan. Include SDOH ICD-10 code. • Select and provide a link to a reading about how SDOH impacts pediatric primary care practice. • In a summary, note major teaching points, avoidance of pitfalls in work-up, defensive practice strategies and interpretation/translation of results. • Submit 3 multiple choice questions related to content (not specifics of the case) with 5 answer choices. One of these questions should incorporate the SDOH addressed in the case.

E = Environmental	S = Social
C = Cultural	P = Policy

	Students will be divided into 10 groups of 2 students each. Each group will have 10 minutes to present their case to the class. Presentation sections will be shared among group members. *The teaching case should come from a real-life case seen by you, your presentation partner or your preceptor. The SDOH you choose may be fictitious but discuss how the chosen SDOH will impact the patient and your management.
Assignment Objectives	

Assignment: Understanding Disparities in Accessing Pain Management
By: Nicholas Giordano

SDOH Pillars Addressed	E ● P
Assignment Type	Research, Interactive
Assignment Details	After reading CDC reports on disparities in the burden of pain and access to pain management nationally, work in small groups to identify 2 to 3 environmental factors, national guidelines, or pieces of legislation that affect the living conditions conducive to explaining why some individuals' or communities' disproportionately experience pain (e.g. expanded access of ACA in certain states, distance to pain specialist in rural communities, etc.)
Assignment Objectives	

Assignment: Impact of SDOH on Validating Classification and Risk Models
By: Melinda Higgins

SDOH Pillars Addressed	Primary: C Secondary: E ● S
Assignment Type	Open Discussion
Assignment Details	Assignment 1: Think about and discuss how various "demographic variables" are contextualized and then operationalized in statistical models. For example, race, which is a non-modifiable variable, is often used as a "risk factor" in many disease models. This may be true when looking at disparities in outcomes. However, race can be operationalized in negative ways. For example, a kidney function status GFR (glomerular filtration rate) is computed using creatine levels and whether someone is African American (AA). AA's "functional status" can sometimes be over-estimated and as a result, some AAs have been penalized and had to wait longer to be put onto a kidney transplant list. Learn more at https://www.kidney.org/atoz/content/race-and-egfr-what-controversy. Assignment 2:

E = Environmental	S = Social
C = Cultural	P = Policy

	Discuss issues related to race and other socio-demographics and their use in training and validating classification and risk models. For example, it is (now) well known that many early facial recognition models did not account for racial and ethnic and even gender variations well due to how the models were originally trained (using mostly White/Caucasian and often male images).

Assignment: An Examination of Environmental Justice
By: Vicki Hertzberg

SDOH Pillars Addressed	E ● S ● P
Assignment Type	Research
Assignment Details	Examination of Environmental Justice - mapping exercise: Overlay maps of Superfund sites vs. average income for census tracts. What is the relationship between the number of Superfund sites in a census tract vs. average income?
Assignment Objectives	

Assignment: Mapping Inequality Redlining in New Deal
By: Lisa Thompson

SDOH Pillars Addressed	E ● S ● C ● P
Assignment Type	Research, Open discussion
Assignment Details	Mapping Inequality Redlining in New Deal America (Created through the collaboration of three teams at four universities) Find where you live in Atlanta: https://dsl.richmond.edu/panorama/redlining/#loc=12/33.794/-84.488&city=atlanta-ga Are you living in a redlined area, as defined by the federal government's Home Owners' Loan Corporation between 1935 and 1940? How was your area defined/described? Areas that received the highest grade of "A"—colored green on the maps—were deemed minimal risks for banks and other mortgage lenders when they were determining who should receive loans and which areas in the city were safe investments. Those receiving the lowest grade of "D," colored red, were considered "hazardous."
Assignment Objectives	

Assignment: Mitigating Impact of Bullying on Mental Health on LGBTQ Youth
By: Philip Davis

SDOH Pillars Addressed	S ● C

E = Environmental	S = Social
C = Cultural	P = Policy

Assignment Type	Research, Writing
Assignment Details	Write an essay discussing an intervention to mitigate the effects of bullying on the mental health of LGBTQ youth and the increased rates of suicide in this community.
Assignment Objectives	

Assignment: Incorporating SDOHs into Clinical Interview
By: Dorothy Jordan

SDOH Pillars Addressed	Primary: E Secondary: S ● C
Assignment Type	Interactive, Writing
Assignment Details	Psychiatric Mental Health Nurse Practitioner Student Assignment
	Clinical Interview
	Assignment: Prepare for a clinical interview as part of your assessment of a seven-year-old patient presenting in the outpatient clinic with sudden onset of selective mutism and school refusal.
	Your seven-year-old patient comes to the clinic accompanied by biological mother and maternal grandmother.
	Submit your clinical interview questions for both the child and parent interviews.
	Highlight the interview questions for your clinical interviews that will assess the environmental pillar of SDOH.
Assignment Objectives	

Assignment: Social Determinants of Health-Based Critique of Measures Used in Research
By: Laura Kimble

SDOH Pillars Addressed	E ● S ● C ● P
Assignment Type	Research, Writing
Assignment Details	Assignment 1: Review instruments/measures used within research studies to examine: 1. Were SDOH considered at all within the research and 2. If SDOH measures were included were important aspects of SDOH included or left out. Assignment 2: Social Determinants of Health-Based Critique of Measures Used in Research

E = Environmental	S = Social
C = Cultural	P = Policy

	Identify 5 quantitative studies in your research area and using the SON SDOH framework identify what pillars were represented in the variables measured, whether SDOH variables were measured with reliable and valid instruments, and propose SDOH variables that should be included in research in their area based on identified gaps.
Assignment Objectives	To critique studies in PhD students' area of research focus for extent to which SDOH variables have been measured and the adequacy of approaches to measurement.

Assignment: Incorporating SDOH Into Lectures and Assignments
By : Lori Modly

SDOH Pillars Addressed	E ● S ● C ● P
Assignment Type	Lecture, Open discussion, Reading, Interactive
Assignment Details	Assignment 1: In considering respiratory, illness care plans, how would SDOH affect a patient's ability to get an inhaler, live in a home free of contaminants, get to the follow-up appointments, access home health, etc. Look at a map of air quality indicators in Metro Atlanta; how does this impact a client's health?

Assignment 2: With regard to vaccines (especially COVID 19), consider the availability, hesitancy, and strategies to combat issues related to these topics. Watch Tyler Perry's video on vaccine hesitancy in the Black community. Then participate in the Emory Vaccine clinic rotating stations through vaccine consent, administering the vaccine, and post-vaccination monitoring. Then fill out a reflection assignment based on your experiences.

Assignment 3: Read and watch the lecture related to Trauma-Informed Care, then read the article on how to provide care to all individuals being mindful of past traumas that may or may not be known. Next, post in the discussion answering how you would respond to one of the various clinical scenarios. You should also review Lindy Grabbe's TIC module & you are encouraged to attend.

Assignment 4: Incorporate the SDOH screening tool developed by CMS and complete the training on how to use the tool. Ask the questionnaire of one of your hospital patients, then discuss the barriers and potential outcomes in post-conference. |
| Assignment Objectives | |

Assignment: Addressing SDOHs in Complex Case Studies
By: Carolyn Reilly

SDOH Pillars Addressed	E ● S ● C ● P
Assignment Type	Interactive, Open Discussion

E = Environmental	S = Social
C = Cultural	P = Policy

Assignment Details	Weekly case study: Break into groups and discuss the 15 questions that guide you through assessment, planning, implementing and evaluating (APIE) care for a specific case study patient. Example: A patient experiencing a Hypertensive Crisis as a multifactorial health situation that can be life threatening. We propose adding additional questions that focus on exploring how the specific 4 pillars of the SDOH framework contribute to the case study. In their small groups, students will discuss the acute and long-term plan of care addressing and mitigating these factors, with specific emphasis on the assessment, treatment, follow-up, and patient education guided by the factors from the SDOH framework. This takes about 45 minutes for the small group. At the end of this time, the class is brought back together, and groups are randomly called to present the answers to the questions. For the specific SDOH question, we will create a grid and solicit 1 unique contributing factor or strategy per group according to APIE based upon the 4 pillars (denoted by 4 different colors). This should result in a student derived, robust picture of how nurses have an opportunity to influence health and wellbeing for complex patients by addressing SDOH factors.
Assignment Objectives	

Assignment: Addressing Racism in Pediatric Practice
By: Imela Reyes

SDOH Pillars Addressed	S
Assignment Type	Open discussion
Assignment Details	Discuss racism in general as a topical discussion and then pull in relevant pediatric points.
Assignment Objectives	

Assignment: Incorporating SDOH Assessment into Windshield Survey
By: Helen Baker

SDOH Pillars Addressed	E ● S ● C ● P
Assignment Type	Research, Writing
Assignment Details	Incorporate SDOH into the windshield survey of the public health nursing course more explicitly. Have each student delve deeper into one aspect of the windshield survey to see how it relates to the SDOH pillars.
Assignment Objectives	

E = Environmental	S = Social
C = Cultural	P = Policy

Assignment: Culturally-Sensitive Risk and Protective Factors for Mental Health
By: Kate Pfeiffer

SDOH Pillars Addressed	Primary: S Secondary: E ● C ● P
Assignment Type	Open discussion
Assignment Details	SDOH and mental health go hand in hand. Facilitate a classroom discussion about culturally sensitive risk factors for mental health (leading to negative outcomes) and protective factors (that can support positive outcomes) that are influenced by social determinants. For example, access to MH services may be considered a privilege afforded to those with economic means. Encouraging students to discuss class, race, social norms, and other social factors' impact on mental health, treatment access, and health outcomes can empower students to address these in individual patient care, and in the broader community.
Assignment Objectives	

Assignment: Addressing SDOHs in SOAP Note
By: Shaquita Starks

SDOH Pillars Addressed	E ● S ● C
Assignment Type	Writing
Assignment Details	Students frequently develop plans without considering SDOH. An example is diet and exercise recommendations. Within their SOAP notes, they should have a section under their plan to address SDOH that may impact adherence to the plan. What grocery stores are proximal to patients' residences? Is there any community center that teaches healthy cooking (culinary med classes)? Are there affordable gyms nearby? Parks, space for walking? Does the patient have dietary restrictions (spiritual) that need to be considered? There are many other questions they can ask, but these are a few ideas.
Assignment Objectives	

Assignment: Understanding Impact of Environmental/Policy Determinants on Patient's Health
By: Linda McCauley

SDOH Pillars Addressed	Primary: E Secondary: P
Assignment Type	Writing
Assignment Details	In this assignment each student will take a patient that they have cared for in the past week and describe environmental factors that could be a determinant in their health and/or disease trajectory. Include the effect of the

E = Environmental	S = Social
C = Cultural	P = Policy

	environmental exposure and the major factors that contribute to the patient's vulnerability.
Assignment Objectives	

Assignment: Access to Resources by Zip Code
By: Susan Brasher

SDOH Pillars Addressed	E ● S
Assignment Type	Research, Writing
Assignment Details	Map the number and degree of quality rated childcare centers in specific zip codes. Then, map the ratings of the school systems in these zip codes. You should be able to see the social environments in which these children reside and the opportunities (or lack thereof) they are afforded, which serves as the foundation of future learning and life success. Consider how you might recommend environmental, social, and policy changes to positively affect these areas.
Assignment Objectives	

Assignment: Clinically Competent and Culturally Proficient Care for Transgender and Gender Nonconforming Patients
By: Elizabeth Downes

SDOH Pillars Addressed	S
Assignment Type	Lecture
Assignment Details	Part 1 of a two-part independent study series entitled Clinically Competent and Culturally Proficient Care for Transgender and Gender Nonconforming Patients.
	Transgender and gender nonconforming people experience high levels of stigma and discrimination in health care. This course gives people who work in health care settings tools that will allow them to better understand their patients' needs so they can provide culturally proficient care to transgender and gender nonconforming patients.
	Describe sex and gender continuums Define terminology used to describe transgender and gender nonconforming people Identify health disparities experienced by transgender and gender nonconforming people
	At the end of the module you will be asked if you want a certificate. Please print or take a screen shot of your request for a certificate. Upload either here.
Assignment Objectives	

E = Environmental	S = Social
C = Cultural	P = Policy

Assignment: Shadowing a Social Worker
By: Suzanne Staebler

SDOH Pillars Addressed	E ● S ● C ● P
Assignment Type	Interactive, Personal Reflection
Assignment Details	Shadow a Social Worker for a day to get a glimpse of the SDOH in real time in our patients. Specific to neonatal, develop a bedside checklist to assess PPD in NICU parents.
Assignment Objectives	

Assignment: Sharing Our Stories
By: Fayron Epps

SDOH Pillars Addressed	C
Assignment Type	Presentation, Open discussion
Assignment Details	Develop a presentation on your culture and present at our routine team meetings. After your presentation, we will have a discussion. This will allow others to further explore and learn about different cultures. This is very important as we go work and recruit from diverse communities.
Assignment Objectives	

Assignment: Health Disparities and Maternal Morbidity
By: Sara Edwards

SDOH Pillars Addressed	E ● S ● C ● P
Assignment Type	Research, Reading, Lecture, Resource
Assignment Details	Text: • Jordan, R. G., Engstrom, J.L., Marfell, J.A., Farley C.L. (2018). Prenatal and Postnatal Care: A Woman-Centered Approach, 2nd edition. Chapter 18. Varney Chapter 3: pp 69-75; 81 Articles: • Alhusen, J. L., Bower, K. M., Epstein, E., & Sharps, P. (2016). Racial Discrimination and Adverse Birth Outcomes: An Integrative Review. Journal of midwifery & women's health, 61(6), 707–720. • Chin, M. H., Clarke, A. R., Nocon, R. S., Casey, A. A., Goddu, A. P., Keesecker, N. M., & Cook, S. C. (2012). A roadmap and best practices for organizations to reduce racial and ethnic disparities in health care. Journal of general internal medicine, 27(8), 992–1000.

E = Environmental	S = Social
C = Cultural	P = Policy

	• Miller, S., Abalos, E., Chamillard, M., Ciapponi, A., Colaci, D., Comandé, D., Diaz, V., Geller, S., Hanson, C., Langer, A., Manuelli, V., Millar, K., Morhason-Bello, I., Castro, C. P., Pileggi, V. N., Robinson, N., Skaer, M., Souza, J. P., Vogel, J. P., & Althabe, F. (2016). Beyond too little, too late and too much, too soon: a pathway towards evidence-based, respectful maternity care worldwide. Lancet (London, England), 388(10056), 2176–2192. • Owens, D. C., & Fett, S. M. (2019). Black Maternal and Infant Health: Historical Legacies of Slavery. American journal of public health, 109(10), 1342–1345. https://doi.org/10.2105/AJPH.2019.305243 • Vedam, S., Stoll, K., Taiwo, T. K., Rubashkin, N., Cheyney, M., Strauss, N., McLemore, M., Cadena, M., Nethery, E., Rushton, E., Schummers, L., Declercq, E., & GVtM-US Steering Council (2019). The Giving Voice to Mothers study: inequity and mistreatment during pregnancy and childbirth in the United States. Reproductive health, 16(1), 77. Active Learning Strategies: • The Lancet Maternal Health https://www.thelancet.com/series/maternal-health-2016 • Complete implicit bias evaluation • https://implicit.harvard.edu/implicit/education.html • Take either the Race IAT or the Skin Tone IAT • There will be an optional Flipgrid for you to discuss your feeling regarding the evaluation here: https://flipgrid.com/4508f4bb Module Resources: • Explore Community organizations, legislation, public health groups involved in maternal mortality: • Black Mamas Matter Alliance https://blackmamasmatter.org/ • Georgia Department of Public Health https://dph.georgia.gov/maternal-mortality • Georgia House of Representatives Study Committee Report: http://www.house.ga.gov/Documents/CommitteeDocuments/2019/MaternalMortality/HR_589_Final_Report.pdf • Georgia Perinatal Quality Collaborative https://georgiapqc.org/
Assignment Objectives	To successfully complete this module, you will be expected to: Identify current international, USA, and Georgia specific data trends and initiatives to address maternal morbidity and mortality Understand the role that implicit bias can play as a strategy in raising awareness as well minimizing unconscious bias in various settings and situations Define the terms: racism, implicit bias, social determinants of health, health disparities, diversity, microaggressions, reproductive justice Explore the concept of respectful maternity care from both a domestic and global perspective Develop skills in the utilization of reflective practice as a mechanism of

E = Environmental	S = Social
C = Cultural	P = Policy

	developing inner wisdom and awareness to engage in meaningful encounters and interactions with others. Develop an awareness of cultural and community involvement/initiatives related to maternal mortality and racial disparities among AA women Engage with midwives involved in both domestic and global work related maternal mortality and health disparities

Assignment: Exploring Racial Disparities in Women's Health Care Group Presentation
By: Trisha Sheridan

SDOH Pillars Addressed	E ● S ● C ● P
Assignment Type	Research, Presentation, Open discussion
Assignment Details	As healthcare providers it is important to acknowledge and examine the effects of racial disparities in women's health care. Black maternal mortality and morbidity has been in the forefront in recent health care crisis. The purpose of this assignment is to delve into the complexities of access and receiving adequate unbiased care.
	The goal is to present one of the many wide-ranging challenges, including but not limited to access to contraception, abortion care to pregnancy, postpartum care/postpartum depression. You will be randomly assigned to a group and together you will need to submit your topic for approval.
	Topics should be specific - not a general overview. Example - topic could be specific to a location - factors in the rate of black maternal mortality and morbidity in Atlanta. Another example could be a presentation on biases in contraception counseling. The presentation needs to include the importance WNHPs have in addressing these concerns as well as local and national resources/programs.
	Feel free to suggest ideas or programs, that could be implemented to help bridge the gap or ameliorate the situation.
	The presentation must include references listed in APA format.
	You have freedom over the design and presentation style.
	Be prepared for meaningful discussion.
Assignment Objectives	

Assignment: Foot Care for the Homeless
By: Rose Murphree

SDOH Pillars Addressed	E ● S ● C ● P
Assignment Type	Interactive, Open Discussion

E = Environmental	S = Social
C = Cultural	P = Policy

Assignment Details	During the upcoming Health Day, you will have the opportunity to volunteer to provide foot care for the homeless. Prior to beginning, we'll discuss the need to pay attention to your own attitudes, beliefs, etc. which may have an influence on your care during the event. After the event, you will be provided with a period for debriefing to discuss any disparities or SDOH issues you may have noticed.
Assignment Objectives	

Assignment: PREPARE Tool for SDOH Assessment
By: Rasheeta Chandler-Coley

SDOH Pillars Addressed	E ● S ● C
Assignment Type	Lecture, Resource
Assignment Details	Use the PRAPARE tool to demonstrate the importance & depth of SDOH assessment that is required by Nurse clinicians, so that we can foster a holistic/equitable approach to care.
Assignment Objectives	

Assignment: SDOH Planning During Patient Discharge
By: Tracey Bell

SDOH Pillars Addressed	E ● S
Assignment Type	Research, Writing
Assignment Details	Write a discharge plan for a patient who had been in the NICU for several weeks. Identify potential social or environmental issues that may impact the infant's long-term outcomes. Once risks are identified, suggest possible community resources available to the family to overcome those proposed barriers.
Assignment Objectives	

Assignment: Understanding Connection Between Food Insecurity and Obesity
By: Amy Becklenberg

SDOH Pillars Addressed	E ● S
Assignment Type	Open discussion, Lecture
Assignment Details	Discuss the connections between food insecurity and obesity. The Food Research and Action Center (FRAC) outlines these connections such as: • Lack of access to healthy, affordable foods (i.e. food desserts) • Fewer opportunities for physical activity • Limited access to health care

E = Environmental	S = Social
C = Cultural	P = Policy

Assignment Objectives	

Assignment: Health Advocacy Assignment
By: Laurie Ray

SDOH Pillars Addressed	P
Assignment Type	Research, Writing
Assignment Details	Reflect on a patient you've seen in clinical whose health or health care was negatively impacted by a policy or law. This may include policies and laws related to: • Access to affordable or universal health insurance • Child or elder protection • Abortion • Guns • Sex work • LGBTQ issues • Education • Housing • Recreational drug use • APRN scope of practice Consider how the policy impacted your patient and how your patient could benefit if the law were amended. For this assignment, you'll be writing an email to one of your elected officials to express your concerns about the law and advocate for change. Depending on whether it is a local, state, or federal law, choose your elected official that has purview over it. You can find all your elected officials by putting in your address here: https://www.commoncause.org/find-your-representative/ This can be especially impactful if there is a current bill under consideration. You will need to reference the specific law or bill in your communication. You can find current legislation in the Georgia General Assembly here: https://www.legis.ga.gov/legislation/all You can find current Georgia code here: http://www.lexisnexis.com/hottopics/gacode/default.asp You can find current legislation at the federal level here: https://www.congress.gov/ And US code here: https://www.govinfo.gov/app/collection/uscode/

E = Environmental	S = Social
C = Cultural	P = Policy

	For helpful tips on writing to your elected officials, check out: https://guides.lib.berkeley.edu/ContactingOfficials/Tips
	Submit the content of your email to canvas.
Assignment Objectives	

Assignment: Nursing Values in Micro-System Assessment
By: Ingrid Duva

SDOH Pillars Addressed	S
Assignment Type	Research, Writing
Assignment Details	Enhance an existing Transforming Healthcare assignment by adding an SDOH lens - for a richer understanding of context. For example, address specifically the "nursing values" when you identify the culture of the unit/clinic etc. Currently, you evaluate context via a micro system assessment (which includes the 5 Ps - purpose, professionals, patients, processes, patterns in addition to identifying communication, and teamwork. Include nursing values noted, in addition to the rest of the cultural conditions, to provide a richer understanding and help predict how and what improvement or change might be most effective.
Assignment Objectives	

Assignment: SDOH Assessment in Ambulatory Care Setting
By: Ingrid Duva

SDOH Pillars Addressed	E ● S ● C ● P
Assignment Type	Research, Writing, Interactive
Assignment Details	Complete an SDOH assessment (considering Environmental, Cultural, Social, and Policy) for your clinical site population - or at least one identified population at that site as part of your QI assignment.
Assignment Objectives	

Assignment: How Geography Impacts Access
By: Bonnie Jennings

SDOH Pillars Addressed	E ● S
Assignment Type	Research, Writing
Assignment Details	Perform an environmental assessment to compare a middle to upper class neighborhood with one where a food desert exists, public transportation is spotty, the crime rate is higher, and kids have more limited access to books and learning.
Assignment Objectives	

E = Environmental	S = Social
C = Cultural	P = Policy

Assignment: Brainstorming Research Topics That Address SDOH of Patient Population
By: Victoria Pak

SDOH Pillars Addressed	E ● S ● C ● P
Assignment Type	Writing
Assignment Details	Discuss how one of the pillars of the SDOH framework impacts the health of the patient/population of interest. Identify how this pillar influences the treatment and outcomes within your population of interest. Think about what future research can be conducted to improve care in the population of your interest.
Assignment Objectives	

Assignment: Holistic Patient Planning Case Study
By: Margaret Conway-Orgel

SDOH Pillars Addressed	E ● S ● C ● P
Assignment Type	Personal reflection, Writing
Assignment Details	You are caring for a former 24-week infant who is now ready to be discharged. The infant is going home in oxygen and will be receiving feeds via G Tube. His mother is a single Black female who is currently working at the Walmart 5 miles from her home. She does not have a car and is dependent on mass transit for transportation. The infant's father is currently incarcerated and will remain so for at least 10 years. Mom moved to the area to follow dad and after he was arrested, found that she was pregnant with their son. She is currently living with her boyfriend's family (grandmother, grandfather and 2 aunts) in a 2-bedroom apartment and is on the list for Section 8 housing however, there is at least a 12 month wait. As part of your role as the APRN caring for this child, it is important that you are: 1. Aware of the 4 aspects of Social Determinants of Health and 2. Based on this knowledge, identify challenges that you anticipate mom will have when she takes her son home and develop an action plan to address at least 2 items in your list of challenges.
Assignment Objectives	

Assignment: Addressing SDOH in Midwifery Case Study
By: Shaquita Starks & Alexis Dunn

SDOH Pillars Addressed	E ● S ● C ● P
Assignment Type	Writing
Assignment Details	Case Study Integrated Behavioral Health APRNs for Mid-Wifery concentration Sharon is a 22-year-old female, who is 5 months pregnant with her second child. She is an unemployed widow, and she and her 4-year-old son now live

E = Environmental	S = Social
C = Cultural	P = Policy

with her older sister, her brother-in-law, and their three children in a two-bedroom apartment. Her husband died last year in a fatal accident on a military base. He was in the Army in good standing. Sharon presents to your clinic with her older sister who brought her in because she has not slept for several days, saying she does not need to sleep, and she has been extremely irritable. Her sister states that whenever they have a conversation, she is extremely talkative, rarely allowing her to get a word in, and is easily distracted. Her sister is also concerned because she is smoking marijuana. During the interview, you also notice that she is constantly talking. Upon further probing about her mood, Sharon tells you, "yeah, about 6 months ago I couldn't stop crying. I just cried and cried for no reason and all I wanted to do was sleep all day." I couldn't concentrate to even making my son food." " I love playing bingo, but I didn't even want to play bingo, so I know something was going on then." The last few days I have gone to bingo every day because I know I am going to win. She was hospitalized one time for an acute psychotic episode after the birth of her first child. She was not able to see her child for several months because he was removed from her custody during her hospitalization and placed in state custody. Despite her history, she says she is not going to take any medicine, saying " I ain't crazy, I pray, and God can fix any problem I have, plus I smoke weed and it calms me down." She adamantly denies any suicidal ideation and denies access to firearms.

- What the most likely diagnosis in this patient?
- How will you approach educating the patient and her sister about her likely condition?
- What questions can you ask to inquire about SDOH to identify community resources and other eligible resources to assist the patient?
- How might you respond to her refusal of medicine and her reliance on prayer and marijuana?
- What first-line medication would you consider if she agrees to take the medication?
- She lacks transportation and does not live near a pharmacy, what steps will you take to assist the patient in acquiring medication?
- What is your medication adherence plan for this patient?
- What safety plan will you create for this patient?
- Considering the patient's history and past circumstances what other questions might you ask?
- What SDOH ICD 10 code might be used in this case?

Assignment Objectives	

Assignment: Reflecting on how SDOH Impact Mental Health Outcomes
By: William Chance Nicholson

SDOH Pillars Addressed	E ● S ● C ● P
Assignment Type	Personal reflection, Writing

E = Environmental	S = Social
C = Cultural	P = Policy

Assignment Details	Activity: Take a few minutes and write down as many things as possible (up to 20) that you feel affect client/patient mental health outcomes in care settings. Then, using the Social Determinants of Health Four Pillar Model, try to assign/arrange these issues into their appropriate pillar. The goal of the exercise is to determine which pillar(s), as a nurse, you identify as bearing the most burden in terms of negative outcomes. This might help inform or shape your practice behaviors or areas where you can affect change as a nurse. Discussions can ensue as to how we help minimize or address these issues utilizing the four-pillar model.
Assignment Objectives	

Assignment: SDOH Influences on the Rate and Causes of Maternal Mortality
By: Wanda Rogler Gibbons

SDOH Pillars Addressed	E ● S ● C ● P
Assignment Type	Open discussion
Assignment Details	Develop a complete patient history (PMH, OB hx, PSH, social, etc), CC(including OLDCARTS), and an exam. When developing care priorities for the patient, focus on one SDOH that influenced this patient's health or care and refer to the evidence to support your proposed plan/intervention. As part of the maternal mortality lecture, discuss the various SDOH influences on the rate and causes of maternal mortality. Think about 1 thing you could do now that could positively influence decreasing maternal mortality.
Assignment Objectives	

Assignment: Impact of SDOH on Health Outcomes of Adult Patients and Veterans
By: Lisa Muirhead

SDOH Pillars Addressed	E ● S ● C ● P
Assignment Type	Personal reflection, Writing
Assignment Details	Use of a case-based exercise that reflects the intersection of SDOH on health outcomes of adult patients and veterans.
Assignment Objectives	

Assignment: Patient Case Study and Presentation
By: Dian Evans

SDOH Pillars Addressed	E ● S ● C ● P
Assignment Type	Presentation, Open discussion
Assignment Details	Topic Presentation Criteria to include 15 minutes with 5 minute Q&A in class presentation and discussion Topic introduction:

E = Environmental	S = Social
C = Cultural	P = Policy

	• Brief overview of epidemiology, pathophysiology and whether the condition is of emerging concern. If there are specific populations most affected, discuss this. If there are any health disparities, discuss. 15%
	Develop a case that helps you illustrate how a patient may present with your topic condition. Include the following: • Chief complaint and HPI along with relevant PMHx, Social Hx, Family Med Hx, ROS • Physical Assessment / Objective Findings • Other relevant Differential Diagnosis • Discussion of relevant diagnostic evaluation and inpatient versus outpatient management. How do you decide?
Assignment Objectives	

Assignment: Trauma Informed Care Discussion
By: Michael Garbett

SDOH Pillars Addressed	S
Assignment Type	Open discussion
Assignment Details	In skills lab students lead a discussion based on Trauma Informed Care based on this article. It addresses the social pillar. https://bit.ly/trauma-informed-np
Assignment Objectives	

Assignment: Advocating to Policy Makers
By: Tova Frenkel

SDOH Pillars Addressed	P
Assignment Type	Research, Writing
Assignment Details	Write a letter to a policy maker (legislator or council member at their local, state, or national level) to promote a policy that addresses and supports the welfare and health of the local community or beyond. Include an evidence summary supporting the request for action.
Assignment Objectives	

Assignment: Capturing SDOHs in Emory EMR
By: Carolyn Clevenger

SDOH Pillars Addressed	E ● S ● C ● P
Assignment Type	Research
Assignment Details	Identify a compatible tool for Emory's electronic medical record to better capture SDOH so that data can be aggregated and correlated with our interventions and outcomes.
Assignment Objectives	

E = Environmental	S = Social
C = Cultural	P = Policy

Assignment: Assessing Racial and Ethnic Disparities in Obstetric Anesthesia
By: Erica Moore

SDOH Pillars Addressed	C
Assignment Type	Research, Writing
Assignment Details	Perform a literature search/review and describe the current issues that affect racial and ethnic disparities in obstetric anesthesia. How does the findings effect the services you provide within the clinical setting?
Assignment Objectives	

Assignment The Role of SDOH in Symptom Management
By: Ethan Cicero

SDOH Pillars Addressed	E ● S ● C ● P
Assignment Type	Research, Presentation, Open Discussion
Assignment Details	Social determinants of health, such as poverty, social isolation, early adversity, and stigma can have a powerful effect on development of symptoms, their nature, chronicity, and how they are measured and managed. Present your research focusing on methods for studying social and structural determinants and to critique literature that specifically looks at symptom-related effects of social factors. Pay particular attention to the different ways in which their moderating versus mediating effects on symptoms can be examined.

In the seminar, we will focus on reviewing, critiquing, and synthesizing current literature and approaches to studying social determinants of health and symptom science broadly.

Discuss theoretical frameworks for understanding the impact of social determinants of health on symptoms. Discuss the utility of theoretical frameworks to study the impact of social determinants of health, which framework(s) may best guide your research, and how is the symptom(s) you are studying are situated within the framework. |
| Assignment Objectives | |

Assignment: SOAP Note with SDOH Planning
By: Jeannie Rodriguez

SDOH Pillars Addressed	E ● S ● C
Assignment Type	Writing
Assignment Details	Obtain a complete health history on your lab partner and document that history in a SOAP note without the O portion, since you have not yet learned the objective components of an exam. Incorporate SDOH in your note, using this as a lens to address any health needs in your plan.
Assignment Objectives	

Assignment: How SDOH Impact maternal mortality in Georgia
By: Priscilla Hall

E = Environmental	S = Social
C = Cultural	P = Policy

SDOH Pillars Addressed	E ● S ● C ● P
Assignment Type	Research, Writing
Assignment Details	Conduct a literature search, using the 4 pillars as a framework, as to what are the SDOH influences over the problem of maternal mortality in Georgia. • As it relates to breastfeeding success • As it relates to preterm birth • As it relates to postpartum depression
Assignment Objectives	

Assignment: SDOH Planning for Surgical Patients
By: Kelly Wiltse-Nicely

SDOH Pillars Addressed	E ● S ● C
Assignment Type	Writing, Open discussion
Assignment Details	The BSN to DNP student, in preparing for their OR cases the next day can consider SDOH in writing their care plan for the day. Further, when reviewing the care plan with their preceptor the next day, they can discuss the SDOH with the preceptor to help foster a culture where SDOH is considered for all patients, all the time. Use the anesthetic care plan format to document subjective and objective findings from patient history and assessment Describe the patient's primary surgical intervention, optimal anesthetic plan, and potential impacts of SDOH on those plans, e.g. social support for post-operative care at home after discharge, recreational drug use, etc. Following discussion with the preceptor, create and implement the anesthetic plan. Note any changes to the plan on the care plan document for easy reference in future cases.
Assignment Objectives	

Assignment: The Accountable Health Communities Health-Related Social Needs Screening Tool
By: Bethany Robertson

SDOH Pillars Addressed	E ● S ● C
Assignment Type	Lecture, Resource
Assignment Details	Use the Accountable Health Communities Health-Related Social Needs Screening Tool produced by CMS to evaluate the health-related social needs of specific populations.
Assignment Objectives	

Assignment: Reading and Reflection: Monique and the Mango Rains
By: Sydney Spangler

SDOH Pillars Addressed	E ● S ● C ● P

E = Environmental	S = Social
C = Cultural	P = Policy

Assignment Type	Reading, Writing
Assignment Details	Monique and the Mango Rains is a story about the experience of an "accidental" midwife in Mali, Monique Dembele, as told by her friend and colleague Kris Holloway, a US Peace Corps Volunteer who was serving in Mali for two years. The book can be found here: https://www.amazon.com/Monique-Mango-Rains-Years-Midwife/dp/1577664353/ref=sr_1_1?ie=UTF8&qid=1544291484&sr=8-1&keywords=monique+and+the+mango+rains Respond to the three items below; EACH of your responses should use complete sentences/well-developed paragraphs and be 250-300 words in length with single-spaced formatting (double spacing between paragraphs). Items 2 and 3 should clearly demonstrate critical thinking and reflect learning from course content. 1. Briefly summarize the major events in the book. 2. Given the context in Mali at the time of the story, what were some significant differences between the lives of Kris and Monique with respect to reproductive health and rights? 3. Do you believe if Kris were pregnant with complications in Mali she would have experienced the same health outcome as Monique? Why or why not?
Assignment Objectives	

Assignment: Racial and/or Ethnic Disparities in Pregnancy
By: Nicole Carlson

SDOH Pillars Addressed	S ● C
Assignment Type	Research, Presentation
Assignment Details	Use a rubric for the upper-level midwifery students for them to benchmark their clinical practice against national statistics on major pregnancy outcomes, then present how outcome statistics differ by client race and ethnicity to identify if there are disparities in existence. This assignment allows students to get experience collecting clinical data for comparison and QI, and also to look for racial and/or ethnic disparities in pregnancy outcomes within the practice.
Assignment Objectives	

Assignment: SDOH Impact on the LGBTQIA+ Population
By: Patricia Moreland

SDOH Pillars Addressed	E ● S ● C ● P
Assignment Type	Lecture, Personal reflection, Writing

E = Environmental	S = Social
C = Cultural	P = Policy

Assignment Details	Lecture on the impact of discrimination, minority stress, policy and laws on LGBTQIA+ health. The concept of intersectionality related to racial, social, and economic factors that impact physical and mental disparities in the LGBTQIA+ population. The role of the nurse in reducing these disparities. Students write a reflection on how SDOH impact the LGBTQIA+ population
Assignment Objectives	

Assignment: Understanding How Health Equity is Addressed in Epidemiological Concepts
By: Ronald Eldridge

SDOH Pillars Addressed	E ● S ● C ● P
Assignment Type	Reading, Research, Writing
Assignment Details	Article review assignment: "Trends in Health Equity in the United States by Race/Ethnicity, Sex, and Income, 1993-2017" • Part A. Discuss the changes in health equity over time as it relates to the Epidemiological concepts of population measures, studies, bias, and causality. • Part B. Choose one of the four SDOH conditions (Social, Environmental, Cultural, Policy) and assess how that SDOH condition may have played a role in the changes (or lack of change) you described in part A.
Assignment Objectives	

Assignment: Discussing SDOH as Part of Pediatric Simulation
By: Jeannie Weston

SDOH Pillars Addressed	S ● C
Assignment Type	Interactive, Open discussion
Assignment Details	• Week 1: Acute illness, and unintentional abuse due to access to informed care • Week 2: Acute and chronic illness and access to informed care including social and cultural differences • Week 3: Acute and chronic illness, substance use with implicit bias, racial disparity and resulting inequity • Week 4: Acute and chronic illness, with disparity in access to care and prenatal education • Week 5: Acute and chronic illness with disparity in education and access to care
Assignment Objectives	• Apply clinical reasoning integrating scientific principles, evidence-based interventions, developmental level and nursing research in planning and evaluating the individualized care of patients with acute and complex alteration in health - this includes patient with disparities in level of education, access to care, language barriers, bias and perception of addiction.

E = Environmental	S = Social
C = Cultural	P = Policy

	• Provide nursing care for patients who are acutely ill based on evidence that contributes to safe and high-quality patient outcomes within the healthcare microsystem. • Demonstrate reflective practice in evaluating personal and professional growth and seek guidance to achieve skill level - students reflect in both prebrief and debrief the problems and discuss and prioritize interventions that patients in each area require for effective care and safe care. • Incorporate bioethical, legal, social, cultural, technological and economic issues in the care of children and adults with acute and complex health problems.

Assignment: How SDOH Contribute to Health Disparities
By: Roxana Chicas

SDOH Pillars Addressed	E ● S ● C ● P
Assignment Type	Research, Writing, Presentation
Assignment Details	Social determinants of health (SDOH) are the conditions in the environments where people are born, live, learn, work, play, worship, and age that affect a wide range of health, functioning, and quality-of-life outcomes and risks (Healthy People 2020). Examples of health disparities: • Black, American Indian, and Alaska Native women are 2-3 times more likely to die from pregnancy related causes than white women https://www.cdc.gov/media/releases/2019/p0905-racial-ethnic-disparities-pregnancy-deaths.html • The rate of preterm birth among Black women (14.4%) is about 50 percent higher than the rate of preterm birth among white women https://www.cdc.gov/reproductivehealth/maternalinfanthealth/pretermbirth.htm • Black women have 2.3 times the infant mortality rate as whites. https://minorityhealth.hhs.gov/omh/browse.aspx?lvl=4&lvlid=23 • Agriculture workers have more than 35 times the risk of heat-related death than workers in all other industries • Gubernot, D. M., Anderson, G. B., & Hunting, K. L. (2015). Characterizing occupational heat-related mortality in the United States, 2000-2010: an analysis using the Census of Fatal Occupational Injuries database. American journal of industrial medicine, 58(2), 203–211. https://doi.org/10.1002/ajim.22381 • Death and hospitalization rates due to COVID-19 disproportionately affect Blacks and Hispanics https://www.cdc.gov/coronavirus/2019-ncov/covid-data/investigations-discovery/hospitalization-death-by-race-ethnicity. • Tribal Communities have 368% greater risk of death related to chronic liver disease compared with to all U.S. races. https://www.ihs.gov/dps/publications/trends2014/

E = Environmental	S = Social
C = Cultural	P = Policy

- LGBTQIA+ youth are 2 to 3 times more likely than non-LGBTQIA+ youth to attempt suicide
https://youth.gov/youth-topics/lgbtq-youth/health-depression-and-suicide
- Justice-involved population is more likely to have high blood pressure than general population
https://www.bjs.gov/content/pub/pdf/mpsfpji1112.
- Risk of childhood lead poisoning is greater in lower-income families
https://ephtracking.cdc.gov/showCommunityDesignAddLinkChildhoodLeadPoisoning.action
- Asthma rates are higher among minority children living in U.S. cities
https://www.aafa.org/asthma-disparities-burden-on-minorities.aspx

Assignment (2-part: Narrative and Concept Map):
For your summative evaluation write a 500-word essay with two references explaining 2-5 SDOH factors that contribute to the health disparity. You may select one health disparity from the list above or identify another.

Describe how SDOH have contributed to the selected health disparity. Include one policy that has influenced the social conditions that generated the health disparity.

Identify the role of one public health core function and one of the ten essential public health services in addressing the selected health disparity.
https://www.cdc.gov/publichealthgateway/publichealthservices/essentialhealthservices.html
Finally, make one community/policy recommendation/intervention that could help close the health disparity gap.

Concept Map: Prepare a stand-alone, concept map that illustrates and clearly links the selected health disparity, at least two (2) SDOH factors, one (1) core function or essential public health service and one (1) policy and show what your recommendations target to help close the health disparity gap. The concept map can be hand-drawn, or you can use any of the online concept-mapping tool, or illustrated on a PowerPoint slide. Be as creative as you would like.

Assignment Objectives	

Assignment: Ambulatory Clinical Debrief
By: Telisa Spikes

SDOH Pillars Addressed	E ● S ● C ● P
Assignment Type	Personal reflection, Writing, Open discussion
Assignment Details	Ambulatory Clinical Debrief
	Reflect back on a patient that you encountered during clinical today with complex medical needs. Identify any barriers the patient may have addressed

E = Environmental	S = Social
C = Cultural	P = Policy

	during the clinical visit that prohibits them from achieving their highest level of health functioning (if applicable) and which pillar does these barriers belong? How can nurses intervene to assist the patient in overcoming these barriers?
Assignment Objectives	

Assignment: Developing Theoretical Framework with SDOH Components
By: Eun-Ok Im

SDOH Pillars Addressed	E ● S ● C ● P
Assignment Type	Writing
Assignment Details	Develop a theoretical framework based on the major concepts of the SDOH framework (e.g., by choosing a specific concept in the frame) that fits with your own phenomenon of interests.
Assignment Objectives	

Assignment: Economic Inequality Map
By: Wonshik Chee

SDOH Pillars Addressed	E ● S
Assignment Type	Research, Writing
Assignment Details	Create an economic inequality map using publicly available information on Internet.
Assignment Objectives	

Assignment: Addressing SDOH in DNP Project Proposal
By: Corrine Abraham

SDOH Pillars Addressed	E ● S ● C ● P
Assignment Type	Research, Resource, Writing
Assignment Details	Outline Discussion: Include potential key discussion point linking key findings to literature/theory, leadership impact or influences, SDH, DEI, and include local/national policy implications and limitations. SDH & Health Equity Module Reading • CDC. (2021). Social Determinants of Health: Know What Affects Health. https://www.cdc.gov/socialdeterminants/index.htm • Rural Health Information Hub. (n.d.).Tools to Assess and Measure Social Determinants of Health. https://www.ruralhealthinfo.org/toolkits/sdoh/4/assessment-tools • Peterson, A., Charles, V., Yeung, D., & Coyle, K. (2020). The Health Equity Framework: A Science- and Justice-Based Model for Public Health

E = Environmental	S = Social
C = Cultural	P = Policy

	Researchers and Practitioners. Health Promotion Practice. 1 - 5. https://doi.org/10.1177/1524839920950730
	• AACN. (2021) The Essentials: Core Competencies for Professional Nursing Education https://www.aacnnursing.org/Portals/42/AcademicNursing/pdf/Essentials-2021.pdf
	• Lingard L. (2015). Joining a conversation: The problem/gap/hook heuristic. Perspectives on Medical Education, 4(5), 252–253. https://doi.org/10.1007/s40037-015-0211-y
	Watch
	• NHWSN. (2020). Integrating Social Determinants of Health into the Nursing Curriculum.
	• IHI. (2019). The Triple Aim and the Social Determinants of Health
	• David R. Williams. (2017). How racism makes us sick
	• IHI. (2016). Does Racism Play a Role in Health Inequities?
	Assignments
	Revised Paper Draft: This semester you will re-format your paper- transitioning from a proposal to a paper/manuscript. Outline/insert implications r/t SDH and DEI as part of the background, methods, or considerations for your discussion/limitations. This will require integration of additional supporting evidence linked specifically to your practice issue as well as concepts included in supplemental resources below.
	Supplemental Resources
	• National Academies of Sciences, Engineering, and Medicine. (2021). The Future of Nursing 2020-2030: Charting a Path to Achieve Health Equity. Washington, DC:The National Academies Press. https://doi.org/10.17226/25982
	• Institute for Healthcare Improvement. (2019). Improving Health Equity: Assessment Tool for Health Care Organizations. Boston, Massachusetts: (Available at www.ihi.org)
	• National Academies of Sciences, Engineering, and Medicine 2017. Communities in Action: Pathways to Health Equity. Washington, DC: The National Academies Press. https://doi.org/10.17226/24624
	• Wyatt, R., Laderman, M., Botwinick, L., Mate, K., & Whittington, J.(2016). Achieving Health Equity: A Guide for Health Care Organizations. IHI White Paper. Cambridge, Massachusetts: Institute for Healthcare Improvement; 2016.
	• Edmunds, M., Bezold, C., Fulwood, C.C., Johnson, B., & Tetteh, H.(2015). The Future of Diversity and Inclusion in Health Services and Policy Research: A Report On The Academy Health Workforce Diversity 2025 Roundtable. https://academyhealth.org/publications/2015-09/future-diversity-and-inclusion-health-services-and-policy-research-report
	• Robin DiAngelo. (2018). Debunking The Most Common Myths White People Tell About Race	Think	NBC News
	• Tyler Merrit. (2018). Before you call.

E = Environmental	S = Social
C = Cultural	P = Policy

Assignment Objectives	• Describe the Emory SON four pillars of SDOH
	• Analyze SDH and DEI influences on a health issue of interest
	• Update your literature review to incorporate SDOH and DEI implications r/t health issue of interest
	• Identify limitations in project methods based on diversity, equity, and inclusivity
	• Describe implications or potential impact of project to address social determinants of health

Assignment: Systems Thinking Approach to address SDOH
By: Susan Swanson

SDOH Pillars Addressed	E ● S ● C ● P
Assignment Type	Interactive, Presentation
Assignment Details	Systems Thinking Approach to address SDOH/Social inequities: Causal Loop Diagram
	Small groups each select one pillar, identify a specific issue within and create causal loop diagram or concept map reflecting some of the many variables and "upstream" drivers contributing to the issue. Present (via Studio or Live Zoom) approaches that may help mitigate one to two of the upstream variables identified. Provide evidence to support initial mapping and proposed "solution". Discuss the role of the DNP in influencing change in this area and how others (studies/evidence) have been successful (or not) in approaching (why/why not)
Assignment Objectives	

Assignment: Ethical Practice in Research Design
By: Drenna Waldrop

SDOH Pillars Addressed	E ● S ● C
Assignment Type	Writing
Assignment Details	Develop a study recruitment plan that addresses how you will engage study participants in ways that are culturally, socially, and economically ethical; that will eliminate coercion, increase access to study benefits to vulnerable and marginalized persons/groups; and will address the lack of trust with medical research.
Assignment Objectives	

Assignment: Care Plan Assignment
By: Nadine Matthie

SDOH Pillars Addressed	E ● S ● C ● P
Assignment Type	Writing
Assignment Details	Care plan assignment: In this assignment, students are presented with a case scenario of a 30-year-old woman being admitted to a telemetry unit with a cardiac diagnosis, altered vital signs, and symptoms of urinary system

E = Environmental	S = Social
C = Cultural	P = Policy

	abnormalities, among other issues. Information is provided regarding physical assessment findings, laboratory values, diagnostic tests, and medications ordered. Based on the details of the case scenario, students are asked to do the following:
	1. Provide a problem list with the 3 most important health problems listed in order of priority (from highest priority to lowest priority).
	2. Provide 1 SMART goal for each item on the problem list (total of 3 SMART goals)
	3. Provide 1 intervention that you will use to achieve each SMART goal (total of 3 interventions).
	While completing this assignment, consider specific SDOH factors that not only influenced the patient's presentation in the scenario but those which can influence the success of the interventions in achieving positive health outcomes.
Assignment Objectives	

Assignment: Impact of SDOH in Data Analysis
By: Sudeshana Paul

SDOH Pillars Addressed	E ● S ● C ● P
Assignment Type	Writing
Assignment Details	Assignment: Examine the resulting data from your research query. Consider the following: • How many variables corresponding to each SDOH pillar were measured in your data? • Based on your data, can you calculate the effect of each SDOH pillar on your outcome of interest? • Would the exposure-outcome relationship differ after you account for variables contributing to each of the SDOH pillar?
Assignment Objectives	

Assignment: Adding SDOH Pillars to Ambulatory Intake Form
By: Sandra Dunbar

SDOH Pillars Addressed	E ● S ● C ● P
Assignment Type	Reading, Research, Writing
Assignment Details	In a class on chronic conditions, and for the clinical module on cardiovascular disease, this assignment will require sharing a clinical intake form, and a literature review. Examine a clinical intake form used in an ambulatory setting that sees persons with coronary artery disease or heart failure. Using the SON Four Pillars of the SDOH framework, what assessment variables would be important to add, and

E = Environmental	S = Social
C = Cultural	P = Policy

	which are incomplete. Document any additional changes from the literature on social determinants of health and cardiovascular disease or equity. This will result in a comprehensive assessment tool; identify what is realistic and feasible to incorporate to guide and improve appropriate and equitable care. Example references: • Havranek EP, Mujahid MS, Barr DA, Blair IV, Cohen MS, Cruz-Flores S, Davey-Smith G, Dennison-Himmelfarb CR, Lauer MS, Lockwood DW, Rosal M, Yancy CW; on behalf of the American Heart Association Council on Quality of Care and Outcomes Research, Council on Epidemiology and Prevention, Council on Cardiovascular and Stroke Nursing, Council on Lifestyle and Cardiometabolic Health, and Stroke Council. Social determinants of risk and outcomes for cardiovascular disease: a scientific statement from the American Heart Association. Circulation. 2015;132:873–898 • O'Neil A, Scovelle AJ, Milner AJ, Kavanagh A. Gender/Sex as a Social Determinant of Cardiovascular Risk. Circulation. 2018 Feb 20;137(8):854-864. doi: 10.1161/CIRCULATIONAHA.117.028595.PMID: 29459471 • Topel, MT, Kelli HM, Lewis TT, Dunbar SB, Vaccarino V. Taylor HA, Quyyumi AA (2018) High neighborhood incarceration rate is associated with cardiometabolic disease in nonincarcerated black individuals, Ann Epidemiology -18 Feb 2. pii: S1047-2797(17)31075-X. doi: 10.1016/j.annepidem.2018.01.011. PMID:29433977
Assignment Objectives	

Assignment: Development of a Centering Pregnancy Module on Maternal Mortality: Focus on Cardiovascular Conditions During Pregnancy
By: Alexis Dunn Amore

SDOH Pillars Addressed	E ● S ● C ● P
Assignment Type	Research, Writing, Interactive
Assignment Details	Development of a Centering Pregnancy Module on Maternal Mortality: Focus on Cardiovascular Conditions During Pregnancy Group Assignment (4 members per group): Develop an educational module about cardiovascular conditions during pregnancy and their association with maternal mortality risk. Incorporate components of each of the 4 SDOH Pillars into the module that will be used to guide the development of a prenatal centering pregnancy group for mothers receiving care at Grady Memorial hospital. For each pillar: 1. Include supporting data/statistics to support the conditions that are selected within each pillar. Present these findings in ways that patients and families can understand 2. Include a list of resources related to each condition 3. Develop a list of culturally appropriate and relevant health promotion

E = Environmental	S = Social
C = Cultural	P = Policy

	activities/interventions that can be incorporated to ameliorate the risk factors for each pillar
Assignment Objectives	

Assignment: Using SDOH Lens to Choose Research Questions
By: Jessica Wells

SDOH Pillars Addressed	E ● S ● C ● P
Assignment Type	Research
Assignment Details	Incorporate an SDOH lens to address your research questions. Instead of focusing on research questions that look at differences on the surface, identify innovative and novel questions that will rectify or mitigate the upstream factors (such as physical, social, economic, and environmental) that are at the root of health disparities.
Assignment Objectives	

Assignment: Live Simulation on Health Equity
By: Quyen Phan

SDOH Pillars Addressed	E ● S ● C ● P
Assignment Type	Interactive, Open discussion
Assignment Details	Participate in a virtual, live simulation on health inequity. Students will be assigned roles, simulating families facing social determinants of health, and at risk for health inequity. All of these are done through Zoom breakout rooms, with pre-brief and debrief, guides attached.
Assignment Objectives	

Assignment: Social and Cultural Considerations in Advance Directive Planning
By: Mellissa Owen

SDOH Pillars Addressed	S ● C
Assignment Type	Personal reflection, Open discussion
Assignment Details	Review the legal Advance Directives document in the state that you want to practice. With this assignment, we talk about several pillars - Social and Cultural being primary. We talk about surrogate decision makers - who is legally the decision maker and the importance of legally defining who they want. We also discuss cultural/spiritual implications related to withholding or withdrawing non beneficial life sustaining therapies.
Assignment Objectives	

Assignment: Examining Social and Environmental Factors That Impact Sleep
By: Glenna Brewster

SDOH Pillars Addressed	E ● S
Assignment Type	Interactive, Research

E = Environmental	S = Social
C = Cultural	P = Policy

Assignment Details	Sleep disturbances is one high priority area for older adults. Address the social and environmental pillars by discussing in groups, reviewing the literature, and interviewing patients on how social factors such as access to healthcare, education and financial resources, and environmental factors like the natural and social environment impact sleep outcomes in older adults. Examine whether there are differences based on race, ethnicity, gender identity, and socioeconomic status.
Assignment Objectives	

Assignment: Medical/Surgical Rotation SDOH Assessment
By: Deborah Michelle Southard-Goodwin

SDOH Pillars Addressed	Primary: C Secondary: E ● S
Assignment Type	Writing, Personal reflection, Open Discussion, Interactive
Assignment Details	During the adult med-surg clinical rotation, students will do a family dynamics, spirituality, and psycho-social assessment on their assigned patient to determine if SDOH are present. The student will initiate a dialog to gather more information and formulate a care plan to address and implement interventions.
Assignment Objectives	

Assignment: SOAP Note: Integrating SDOH Into Planning
By: Priya Schaffner

SDOH Pillars Addressed	E ● S ● C
Assignment Type	Writing
Assignment Details	Develop a SOAP note that includes an assessment/plan that addresses each of the four SDOH pillars.
Assignment Objectives	

E = Environmental	S = Social
C = Cultural	P = Policy

References

1. Rosenshine B. Principle of instruction. International Academy of Education, UNESCO. Geneva: International Bureau of Education; 2010. Available from www.ibe.unesco.org/fileadmin/user_upload/publications/educational_practices/edpractices_21.pdf
2. Maehr M, Meyer H. Understanding motivation and schooling: where we've been, where we are, and where we need to go. Educ Psychol Rev. 1997;9:371–409.
3. Svinicki MD. Learning and motivation in the postsecondary classroom. Bolton, MA: Anker; 2004.

4. Artiga S, Hinton E. Beyond health care: the role of social determinants in promoting health and health equity what are social determinants of health. Focus on Health in Non-Health Sectors. 2018;1–23.
5. Freire P. Pedagogy of the oppressed. New York: Continuum; 1970.
6. Sharma M, Pinto AD, Kumagai AK. Teaching the social determinants of health: a path to equity or a road to nowhere? Acad Med. 2018;93(1):25–30. https://doi.org/10.1097/ACM.0000000000001689.
7. Naegle MA, Finnell DS, Kaplan L, Herr K, Ricciardi R, Reuter-Rice K, Oerther S, Van Hook P. Opioid crisis through the lens of social justice. Nurs Outlook. 2020;68(5):678–81. https://doi.org/10.1016/j.outlook.2020.08.014.
8. Duque RB. Black health matters too… especially in the era of Covid-19: how poverty and race converge to reduce access to quality housing, safe neighborhoods, and health and wellness Services and increase the risk of co-morbidities associated with global pandemics. J Racial Ethn Health Disparities. 2021;8(4):1012–25. https://doi.org/10.1007/s40615-020-00857-w.

Curriculum Mapping: Integrating Social Determinants of Health Within Nursing Education

4

Autherine Abiri, Wanjira Kinuthia, and Elizabeth Downes

Learning Objectives

- Understand the need and relevance of SDOH integration within nursing education.
- Define curriculum mapping.
- Describe the steps included in the Five-Step Mapping Process for integrating SDOH within nursing education.
- Develop curriculum mapping skills to integrate SDOH content within an individual course and curriculum.

Introduction

Social determinants of health (SDOH) are the conditions and systems of influence that impact health outcomes [1, 2]. The World Health Organization further identifies these as nonmedical factors that influence health outcomes and equity; they are the circumstances in which people are born, grow, work, live, and age. SDOH are the broader forces, economic policies and systems, development agendas, social norms, social policies, and equities, which shape the conditions of daily life [1]. Collectively, these influences include social, economic, environmental, cultural, and political factors that shape the conditions of everyday life for all patients. The substantial ability of SDOH to shape health outcomes renders it as a significant element for exploring health inequities. Moreover, this calls for the nursing profession to address SDOH, not only at the bedside, but to ensure the inclusion of SDOH within nursing education.

To effectively address existing inequities within healthcare, we must strengthen the inclusion of SDOH within nursing curricula. There is insufficient integration of

A. Abiri (✉) · W. Kinuthia · E. Downes
Nell Hodgson Woodruff School of Nursing, Emory University, Atlanta, GA, USA
e-mail: Autherine.abiri@emoryhealthcare.org; wkinuth@emory.edu; edownes@emory.edu

SDOH within nursing education [3]. The comprehensive incorporation of SDOH throughout nursing curricula ensures that we have a nursing workforce prepared to build a healthy population [4]. With their strategic positioning on the frontline of healthcare, nurses recognize the influence that SDOH may have on the overall wellness of individuals and populations. Nursing roles vary from delivering care in hospitals to shaping public policy, which in turn can impact the health of individuals and communities. These roles place nurses in the unique position to improve health outcomes by being prepared to address healthcare disparities and inequities that impact society. Thus, integration of SDOH has been recognized as a vital component of nursing education [5].

As noted in previous chapters, the NHWSN *Four Pillars of SDOH* organizes SDOH into four general domains: Social, Environmental, Cultural, and Political (see Fig. 4.3). Understanding SDOH, and the effect it has on health outcomes should be integrated into all levels of nursing education. The pillars can be introduced at the beginning of the nursing education journey and remain a priority in clinical experiences where students can incorporate the SDOH pillars into comprehensive care plans [6].

Curriculum Mapping Defined

Curriculum mapping is the systematic method for identifying and linking student outcomes and curriculum learning activities. It is used to map learning outcomes throughout a single course or across programs of study, map course progression, track and evaluate both the teaching and assessment of student learning outcomes and detect learning gaps [7]. Although there are various course and improvement strategies that faculty and administration apply, processes involve a feedback loop based on learning outcomes and learner and instructor feedback, and it requires ongoing monitoring and review of the courses [7].

Curriculum mapping is a versatile process tool that can help faculty determine whether different course components align and what adjustments should be made. Process mapping has the advantage of representing spatially the different components of the curriculum so that the big picture, the relationships, and connections between the parts of the map are easily recognizable. This visual representation is more meaningful to the course developer, instructor, and students [7, 8], and helps guide program design and improvement, consistency, fairness, quality, cohesion, and effectiveness [7].

Curriculum mapping can be used for different purposes, including examining a curriculum at its planning and design stage, refining it or evaluating an existing curriculum's effectiveness [7]. This discussion pertains to evaluating an existing curriculum to determine how social determinants of health are integrated into course design and delivery. We combine curriculum mapping and pedagogical methods to create a step-by-step framework that guides the comprehensive inclusion of SDOH within pre- and post-licensure nursing programs. This continuous improvement of teaching and learning is critical for any institution of higher education. This is particularly important when aiming to meet accreditation standards and ensure accountability by all stakeholders [8].

Curriculum Mapping Process

The curriculum mapping process involves integrating SDOH pillars and learning topics throughout pre- and post-licensure nursing programs. The goal of integration is to move away from the pattern of having single lectures or assignments on SDOH only seen in a limited number of courses, and to shift to a more comprehensive approach that fully integrates SDOH within nursing education. Data from the curriculum mapping process allows one to see the relative contributions of each individual course and how SDOH topics are strategically woven throughout pre- and post-licensure courses. Additionally, curriculum mapping makes it possible to see the process used to evaluate the curriculum and the rationale that guides changes within the curriculum in an effort toward achieving continuous quality improvement for the courses and the programs [9].

The methodological approach for integrating SDOH throughout pre- and post-licensure nursing programs occurs in a five-step process developed by a subcommittee of the Nell Hodgson Woodruff School of Nursing's (SON's) curriculum committee. This innovative SDOH curriculum mapping process includes five steps:

Step 1. Establish SDOH learning goals, objectives, and outcomes.
Step 2. Create a baseline curriculum map.
Step 3. Implement individual course analysis.
Step 4. Build an integrative and comprehensive map.
Step 5. Review for ongoing sustainability.

Figure 4.1 is an illustration that outlines the *Five-Step Process for Curriculum Mapping of SDOH*, and Fig. 4.2 is a timeline of events to facilitate effective completion of the mapping process. In the following sections we explain in detail each step of the mapping process.

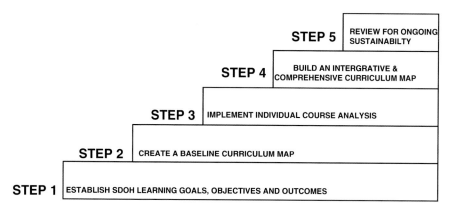

Fig. 4.1 Five-step process for curriculum mapping of SDOH

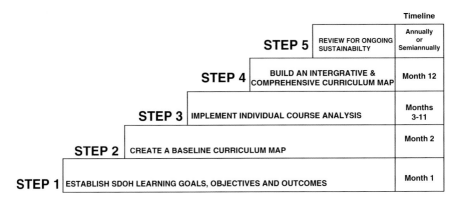

Fig. 4.2 Five-step process for curriculum mapping of SDOH with a timeline

Table 4.1 SDOH learning objectives

Program of study	Objective
Pre-licensure	Students will *define and/or assess* the influences of SDOH (cultural, social, environmental, and political) on illness and wellness in healthcare at the individual, family, community, and societal levels
Post-licensure	Students will *evaluate and apply* evidence-based knowledge about the influences of SDOH (cultural, social, environmental, and political) on illness and wellness related to advanced practice and research with diverse populations at the individual, family, community, and societal levels

Step 1: Establish SDOH Learning Goals, Objectives, and Outcomes

To initiate the process of integrating SDOH throughout nursing curricula, a curriculum mapping committee must first be established and led by a faculty member who will oversee and chair the process. An ideal mapping team will include faculty that serve on the school's curriculum committee. Committee members should also include individuals who are experts on instructional design. The shared vision of the mapping committee is to integrate all four SDOH pillars throughout every course within the curriculum. For this to become effective, the mapping team will develop SDOH learning goals, objectives, and outcomes for pre- and post-licensure nursing programs. Table 4.1 includes examples of pre- and post-licensure SDOH objectives using Bloom's Taxonomy.

- Pre-licensure objectives: Students will define and/or assess the influences of SDOH (cultural, social, environmental, and political) on illness and wellness in healthcare at the individual, family, community, and societal levels.
- Post-licensure objectives: Students will evaluate and apply evidence-based knowledge about the influences of SDOH (cultural, social, environmental, and political) on illness and wellness related to advanced practice and research with diverse populations at the individual, family, community, and societal levels.

Step 2: Create a Baseline Curriculum Map

Following committee approval of SDOH learning goals, objectives, and outcomes, the SDOH mapping team will create a baseline curriculum map for undergraduate and graduate nursing programs. This initial map will capture the initial status of the inclusion of SDOH throughout each program of study. Baseline curriculum map headings reflect course learning objectives and activities in relation to SDOH pillars. Table 4.2 is a template baseline map with headings and course examples.

Table 4.2 SDOH curriculum baseline map with examples

Course title	Describe what you do in your course related to SDOH	SDOH pillar(s) for course	Student learning activities	Weekly objectives for activities
Advanced Health Assessment	A. Clinically Competent and Culturally Proficient Care for Transgender and "Gender Nonconforming Patients" Parts 1 and 2 B. Assess how patients prefer to make medical decisions— individually, as a family, or through a specific authority figure	Social conditions Cultural conditions Policies/Laws	A. Complete modules for certificate; content on exams B. Discussion	A. Part 1: • Describe sex and gender continuums • Define terminology used to describe transgender and gender nonconforming people • Identify health disparities experienced by transgender and gender nonconforming people A. Part 2: • Describe accepted medical protocols for gender affirmation • Describe models of informed consent for gender affirmation • Determine which primary care services to provide to patients of any gender identity based on their anatomy and physiology B. Discuss how culture influences the way patients and families discuss medical information and make medical decisions

(continued)

Table 4.2 (continued)

Course title	Describe what you do in your course related to SDOH	SDOH pillar(s) for course	Student learning activities	Weekly objectives for activities
Staying Healthy in Pediatrics	Health disparities across groups based on racism and bias, including LGBTQ+	Policy	Adverse Childhood Events and Trauma Informed Care, Successful transition of care for cognitively impaired/autistic children; open discussion re: healthcare disparities *d/t* racism and other biases; GDOH: Children First/ Babies Can't Wait	Critique and respond to policies that influence healthcare delivery systems and impact preventive healthcare
Pediatric Wellness	SDOH module covering structural racism and health disparities	Social Environmental Policy	Lecture format class	Course objective: Evaluate psychosocial, biological, environmental, spiritual, cultural, and competing factors that influence adoption of healthy lifestyle practices and health status. Module Objectives: Describe the extent of the challenges of child and family poverty Understand the relationship between health status and biology, individual behavior, health services, social factors, and policies Emphasize an ecological approach to disease prevention and health promotion Understand the fundamentals of the ecological approach on both individual- and population-level determinants of health and interventions

Table 4.3   Example of individual course analysis

Course name: Advanced Health Assessment				
Assessment (title)	Type	Level	SDOH pillar	Assignment information/ SDOH content covered
SDOH	Discussion	Intermediate	Social, cultural, environmental, policy/law	Students post an analysis about how SDOH affects COVID-19 testing, vaccination, or treatment
Professional Nursing Topic Paper	Assignment	Advanced	Social, cultural, environmental, policy/law	Students explore issues relevant to professional nursing
LGBTQIA+ Simulation	Case study	Advanced	Social, cultural	Students respond to video case studies and simulations on LGBTQIA+

This map serves as the starting point for comparison during the SDOH mapping process. It is especially useful for identifying overlapping elements and existing gaps for SDOH integration within each course. To complete this baseline curriculum map, all faculty in the pre- and post-licensure programs should enter their individual course content on the map under each appropriate column heading (see Table 4.3). This can be accomplished with the use of a shared digital filing system. An alternative is to have the curriculum mapping team representative meet with each course coordinator to determine the relevant content.

Regardless of which alternative is used, involving all faculty within this mapping step is critical and requires a systematic approach that incorporates effective communication. Communication regarding the mapping process should be initiated with an informative meeting inviting all faculty. During this meeting, the shared vision of SDOH integration along with the mapping process will be communicated. This baseline map should be completed in an organized and scheduled manner that allows faculty sufficient time and flexibility to thoroughly assess their course content in relation to the SDOH pillars. The timeframe for the completion of this baseline map following the informative meeting may vary and is dependent upon faculty participation. Program directors are especially encouraged to help facilitate this process in coordination with the mapping committee. By engaging program directors, the mapping team establishes an effective and efficient connection with all faculty. With ample faculty engagement, the anticipated timeframe for baseline map completion is within a 1-month period following the informative meeting.

Step 3: Implement Individual Course Analysis

Once the baseline map is completed, the mapping team begins the process of individual course analysis. Each course is individually explored for their inclusion of SDOH pillars within their learning objectives, activities, and assessment tools. This step of the mapping process is an in-depth review that serves to assess the quality of

SDOH integration within each course. Individual course review and analysis are guided by the following questions:

1. Does the course contain learning outcomes that are linked to the competencies and content areas in SDOH pillars?
2. If so, at what level on Bloom's Taxonomy? At what depth did each course address SDOH competencies and content areas?
3. Holistically (programmatically), do the courses interact or align to address specific SDOH competencies and content areas? To what extent was the specific course objective in the syllabus addressed in the course content and in the assignments? See Table 4.1 for pre- and post-licensure objectives.
4. Were additional learning outcomes specific to SDOH pillars integrated into the course? If so, to what extent were they aligned with the assignments? At what level on Bloom's Taxonomy?

This review encompasses all didactic courses and does not include labs and clinical/practicum courses, as they are separate from didactic courses in our curriculum. Each course is reviewed using a two-phase qualitative and quantitative approach. The first phase, a qualitative holistic review, scans course syllabi and course content broadly to determine if and how SDOH pillars are included in the courses from an instructional and learning activity perspective. The analysis also looks at whether course and module learning outcomes are aligned with assignments. The metrics are course artifacts, for example, textbook chapters, PowerPoint slides, recorded video lectures, case studies, empirical articles, papers, policy papers, and instructional videos. The initial part of the individual course analysis is conducted by the mapping team using the Learning Management System (LMS) course sites as an inventory. Information for each course to review is gathered using the SON's online LMS (i.e., course Canvas). Once again, the timeline needed to conduct this should allow for ample review. The mapping committee may need to elicit additional assistance from faculty members to complete it in an organized fashion. Additionally, this may be contracted out to qualified individuals in instructional design. It may require as many as 8 months to complete.

Using a matrix (Fig. 4.3), the second phase entails an in-depth analysis of how the assignments addressed SDOH pillars. This quantitative phase documents the number of assignments that specifically integrate SDOH pillars. The levels of the assignments are categorized based on Bloom's Taxonomy, i.e., foundational (remembering and understanding), intermediate (applying and analyzing), and advanced (evaluating and creating) [10, 11]. The types of assignments including quizzes, forum discussions, case studies, video analyses, presentations, and policy briefs, are noted in the curriculum mapping matrix. The in-depth assignment review also identifies which pillars are embedded in the assignments. Using the matrix as a template and guide, this quantitative approach should occur simultaneously with this qualitative approach.

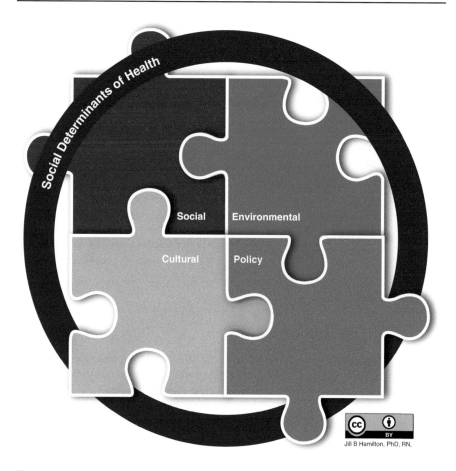

Fig. 4.3 NHWSN School of Nursing Four-Pillar SDOH framework

Step 4: Build an Integrative and Comprehensive Map

Once each course is analyzed, the next step is to build an integrative comprehensive curriculum map for each program of study that incorporates the four pillars of SDOH. The goal of this map is to effectively represent the integration of all four SDOH pillars throughout all pre- and post-licensure programs. The mapping template is similar to the baseline map and contains the same format and headings, thus allowing a direct comparison. With a comprehensive map for each program of study, the mapping team searches for redundancies and gaps across all programs. At this point, improvement should be noted regarding the elimination of gaps and redundancies when compared to the initial baseline map.

Step 5: Review for Ongoing Sustainability

Maintaining a sustainable mapping process is imperative for preserving the inclusion of SDOH within the curricula. A dedicated review committee should be established within the curriculum committee to systematically approach this review process and maintain updates. There should be a periodic ongoing review of learning objectives, outcomes, and activities for each course and across all programs of study. Once each program has a comprehensive SDOH map, the ongoing review is initially recommended on a semester-by-semester basis. Eventually, a curriculum mapping review of learning objectives, outcomes, and activities should be conducted annually/semiannually as part of the course evaluation process and incorporated into the Systematic Review Plan. During each review period, learning goals, objectives and outcomes should be reviewed for any updates and modifications to represent current topics. The committee reviews if course assignments incorporated SDOH concepts in meaningful and practical ways. This was done to determine if exposure to SDOH in a particular course reading, a PowerPoint slide or video was introduced and, if it achieved the next level, how these determinants play a role in health. Exemplars of assignments are given in Chap. 5.

Summary

Curriculum mapping is a dynamic process that effectively captures the expanding nature of SDOH integration within both undergraduate and graduate nursing curricula. Although this process is complex and time consuming, implementing a systematic approach provides useful results in which faculty can identify gaps and redundancies of SDOH throughout pre- and post-licensure curricula. SDOH curriculum mapping is a necessary tool for nursing faculty to utilize, build, modify, and integrate courses that accurately reflect SDOH intersections. The integration of SDOH within nursing curricula ensures that we build global nurses ready to provide patient-centered care. It is also essential to revisit courses and check for "drift" and engage faculty in regular dialogs about the purpose and value of including SDOH pillars in the courses. Ultimately, when students graduate, they will be better prepared to address the situations while providing quality healthcare. Periodic mapping will also allow the curriculum to remain relevant and current by broadening faculty members' knowledge on how the pillars can be an integral part of the School of Nursing's curriculum. This can be done by updating the instructional resources and learning strategies that best expose students to the pillars in a manner that raises their awareness of social determinants of health and how they impact their patients.

Reflections

- The curriculum mapping process requires engaging key stakeholders which include developing partnerships with faculty, leadership, and students.
- Threading SDOH within each course and across all programs of study is a complex process that requires ongoing revisions for sustainability.
- A dedicated mapping committee is necessary to maintain ongoing progress.

Chapter Review Questions

1. What is curriculum mapping?
   (a) A process for examining and connecting student outcomes and curriculum learning activities.
   (b) A process that identifies learning outcomes throughout a single course or across programs of study.
   (c) A process that is used to identify curriculum gaps and redundancies.
   (d) All of the above.
2. What is the significance of an individual course analysis, the third step of SDOH curriculum mapping?
   (a) An in-depth review that evaluates the integration of SDOH pillars within a course's learning objectives, activities, and assessment tool.
   (b) Includes labs and clinical practicum courses.
   (c) Does not integrate Bloom's taxonomy.
   (d) All of the above.
3. The purpose of having a baseline map and a comprehensive integrative map is to
   (a) Map SDOH redundancies and gaps.
   (b) Compare and evaluate the progression of SDOH integration.
   (c) Prepare students to assess and address SDOH.
   (d) All of the above.

   Answers
- 1. (d), 2. (a), 3. (d)

References

1. World Health Organization. Social determinants of health. 2022. https://www.who.int/health-topics/social-determinants-of-health#tab=tab_1. Accessed 29 Sept 2022.
2. Centers for Disease Control and Prevention. Healthy people 2020. https://www.cdc.gov/nchs/healthy_people/hp2020.htm. Accessed 3 Oct 2022.
3. Tilden VP, Cox KS, Moore JE, Naylor MD. Strategic partnerships to address adverse social determinants of health: redefining health care. Nurs Outlook. 2018;66:233–6.
4. A vision for integration of the Social Determinants of Health into Nursing Education Curricula. 2019. https://www.nln.org/docs/default-source/uploadedfiles/default-document-library/social-determinants-of-health.pdf?sfvrsn=aa66a50d_0. Accessed 3 Oct 2022.
5. Porter K, Jackson G, Clark R, Waller M, Stanfill AG. Applying social determinants of health to nursing education using a concept-based approach. J Nurs Educ. 2020;59:293–6.
6. Mahony D, Jones EJ. Social determinants of health in nursing education, research, and health policy. Nurs Sci Q. 2013;26:280–4.
7. Kopera-Frye K, Mahaffy J, Svare GM. The map to curriculum alignment and improvement. Collect Essays Learn Teach. 2008;1:1–8.
8. Levin PF, Suhayda R. Transitioning to the DNP: ensuring integrity of the curriculum through curriculum mapping. Nurs Educ. 2018;43:112–4.
9. Perlin MS. Curriculum mapping for program evaluation and CAHME accreditation. J Health Admin Educ. 2011;28:27–47.
10. Bloom BS. Taxonomy of educational objectives: the classification of educational goals. 2nd ed. Addison Wesley Longman; 1956.
11. Krathwohl DR. A revision of Bloom's taxonomy: an overview. Theory Pract. 2002;41:212–8.

SDOH in Action: Exemplars of Incorporating SDOH Content in Entry-Level and Advanced-Level Nursing Education

5

Beth Ann Swan, Lalita Kaligotla, Autherine Abiri, Lindsey Allen, Amy Becklenberg, Christina K. Bhatia, Sofia Biller, Susan Brasher, Rasheeta Chandler, DeJuan Charles, Erica Davis, Anneke Demmink, Harrison Boyd Diamond, Elizabeth Downes, Rebekah Elting, Wendy R. Gibbons, Nicholas A. Giordano, Jill B. Hamilton, Caroline Kee, Stephanie Lee, Alyssa Meadows, Lori A. Modly, Kenneth Mueller, Caitlyn Plattel, Melissa Poole-Dubin, Maria-Bernarda Saavedra, Isake Slaughter, Shaquita Starks, Susan L. Swanson, Isabella Upchurch, Jessica Wells, Phyllis Wright, and Irene Yang

B. A. Swan (✉) · L. Kaligotla · A. Abiri · L. Allen · A. Becklenberg · C. K. Bhatia · S. Biller ·
S. Brasher · R. Chandler · D. Charles · E. Davis · A. Demmink · H. B. Diamond · E. Downes ·
R. Elting · W. R. Gibbons · N. A. Giordano · J. B. Hamilton · C. Kee · S. Lee · A. Meadows ·
L. A. Modly · K. Mueller · C. Plattel · M. Poole-Dubin · M.-B. Saavedra · I. Slaughter ·
S. Starks · S. L. Swanson · I. Upchurch · J. Wells · P. Wright · I. Yang
Nell Hodgson Woodruff School of Nursing, Emory University, Atlanta, GA, USA
e-mail: beth.ann.swan@emory.edu; lalita.kaligotla@emory.edu; Autherine.abiri@emory-
healthcare.org; Lindsey.allen2@emory.edu; amy.becklenberg@emory.edu; ckbhati@emory.
edu; sofia.biller@emory.edu; susan.n.brasher@emory.edu; r.d.chandler@emory.edu;
endavi5@emory.edu; anneke.demmink@emory.edu; edownes@emory.edu; Rebekah.elting@
emory.edu; wgibbon@emory.edu; nicholas.a.giordano@emory.edu; jbhamil@emory.edu;
ckee@emory.edu; Stephanie.m.lee@emory.edu; Alyssa.meadows@emory.edu; lori.a.modly@
emory.edu; kjmuell@emory.edu; Caitlyn.Plattel@emory.edu; melissa.a.poole@emory.edu;
maria-bernarda.saavedra@emory.edu; Isake.Slaughter@emory.edu; shaquita.starks@emory.
edu; susan.lynn.swanson@emory.edu; isabella.upchurch@emory.edu; jholme3@emory.edu;
Phyllis.p.wright@emory.edu; irene.yang@emory.edu

Learning Objectives for the Chapter

1. Discuss the importance of social determinants of health (SDOH) in nursing education.
2. Describe a framework for entry- and advanced-level professional nursing education informed through an SDOH lens.
3. Apply the SDOH framework to course activities and assignments.
4. Consider SDOH content across pre- and post-licensure courses.

Introduction

Thus far, readers have been provided with the history of SDOH, a framework for guiding the exploration of SDOH in education, along with faculty and student resources, and curriculum mapping. This chapter focuses on application, action-oriented teaching learning examples for entry-level professional nursing education and advanced-level nursing education. Each exemplar describes the background and course objectives focused on the SDOH, a course description is provided along with the course assignment, and student and/or faculty reflections on the SDOH-focused assignment. The course descriptions and assignment exemplars are informed by the American Association of Colleges of Nursing's (AACN) *The Essentials: Core Competencies for Professional Nursing Education* [1]. Core domains, concepts, and competencies for professional nursing education are examined within a SDOH lens as illustrated in Fig. 5.1.

Seven entry-level course exemplars are included: pediatric nursing, mental health nursing, pharmacology for nursing practice, art and science of nursing practice,

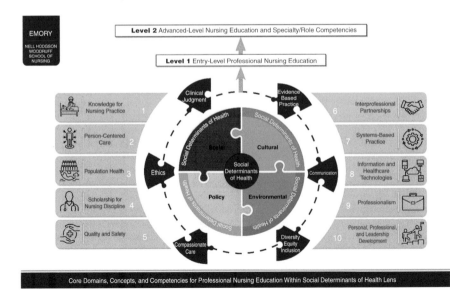

Fig. 5.1 Core domains, concepts, and competencies for professional nursing education within social determinants of health lens

social responsibility and ethics, evidence-based practice for the professional nurse, and nursing honors course. Three advanced-level course exemplars are included: advanced health assessment (MSN), omics in health and disease (PhD), analysis of complex systems for populations and organizations (DNP), and an SDOH application-focused DNP scholarly project. The chapter concludes with a SDOH simulation exemplar focused on compassionate care and respectful communication.

Entry-Level Professional Nursing Education Exemplars

Pediatric Nursing

Susan Brasher and Anneke Demmink

Background

Person and family-centered care is increasingly becoming a prominent model to structure family involvement in pediatric care [2]. The SDOH framework considers the impact of surrounding conditions and wider set of forces and systems on a person's health and outcomes [3]. Similarly, a person- and family-centered approach places greater emphasis on collaborating with the whole family in consideration of the surrounding influences and their impact on promoting the health and wellbeing of children [4]. This type of model redefines traditional relationships within healthcare settings to collaborate with children and families as allies to enhance health outcomes and improve patient and family experiences of care [4]. Using a person- and family-centered care approach, nurses are poised to deliver effective care tailored to the major influences surrounding children, including the SDOH. Furthermore, this curricular framework directly aligns with the Robert Wood Johnson Foundation [5] and National League for Nursing [6] recommendations for nursing programs to better incorporate population-focused competencies to better prepare nurses to meet the complex needs of patient populations, and to integrate the SDOH more fully into nursing curricula.

Nurses play a pivotal role in providing strategies to combat the negative health outcomes associated with SDOH. For this reason, it is crucial to incorporate SDOH into nursing curricula to better prepare those entering the nursing profession. However, schools of nursing often lack faculty-led discussions on current civic events and intentional curricular efforts to address SDOH and downstream effects on health and health outcomes [7]. According to Thornton and Persaud [8], it is important to integrate SDOH concepts throughout nursing curricula rather than in a sporadic and isolated manner. Such intentionality in education is required to best prepare the nursing workforce to address SDOH and close gaps in healthcare access and address disparities in health outcomes [9]. This pedagogical exemplar highlights the full integration of SDOH into a pediatric pre-licensure nursing course through a person- and family-centered care approach.

Course Description

NRSG 328 This course aims to facilitate student learning and acquisition of clinical judgment skills necessary to provide person- and family-centered care that addresses the unique responses of children and their families to acute and chronic illness. Emphasis is placed on health teaching, promotion, restoration, and health maintenance needs of children and their families. Students explored the influences of SDOH (cultural, social, environmental, and political) on pediatric illness and wellness.

AACN Essentials Domain 1: Knowledge for Nursing Practice, Domain 2: Person-Centered Care, Domain 7: Systems-Based Practice

Description of Course Activities and Assignments

The primary means of evaluation for this course were objective examinations. A total of three exams were administered during the course, including a cumulative final exam. Each exam included opportunities for students to identify ways SDOH impact various aspects of a pediatric patient's health and health outcomes. Exam questions on this content include case study, fill in the blanks, and essay questions.

Weekly classroom discussions explored pediatric health and health outcomes in the context of their family and surrounding influences. Each week, students were expected to identify the complicated ways in which SDOH influences pediatric health and health outcomes, as well as ways to address SDOH through a person- and family-centered approach. Through intentional, frequent exposure to SDOH in the pediatric course, students were able to apply these concepts across different contexts (e.g., primary care, acute care, and community settings).

Weekly discussions were based on the NHWSN SDOH four-pillar framework (e.g., social, cultural, environmental, and policy). Topics were addressed from a Bloom's hierarchical pedagogical approach to guide the learners from the beginning stages of knowledge and comprehension, followed by application and analysis, resulting in synthesis and evaluation as a precursor to successfully translate knowledge and skills to practice. In-class activities were provided to students to create an open dialogue on the impact SDOH has on pediatric health and health outcomes. Examples of in-class activities include:

1. Provide a tailored plan of care in consideration of social and cultural factors for nutritional approaches of infants.
2. Map the number and degree of quality rated childcare centers in specific zip codes. Then, map the ratings of the school systems in these zip codes. Consider the social environments in which children reside and the opportunities (or lack thereof) they are afforded, which serve as the foundation of future learning and life success. Consider how social, cultural, environmental, and policy changes positively influence children and families residing in these areas.

Student Assignment Exemplars

Exam questions were developed to gauge student knowledge on the impact of SDOH on children and families. Examples of exam questions include:

1. Identify social determinants of vaccine hesitancy.
2. Describe the impact SDOH has on pediatric hospitalizations, including disparate health outcomes and the parent's ability to be present during hospitalization.

3. Consider how SDOH impacts hospital discharge planning and ways to work with children and families to improve transition of care.
4. Explore the impact of access to necessary services for the treatment and prevention of common pediatric conditions.

Reflection: Faculty

Intentional incorporation of SDOH within a pediatric nursing course provides faculty an opportunity to highlight the ways in which SDOH impacts children across conditions, settings (e.g., community and hospital), and lifespan. Considering the ways SDOH impacts children within the larger context of the family, community, and systems they navigate from a person- and family-centered care approach is paramount. Too often care is provided without regard to these important contexts, which further contributes to poorer health and health outcomes for pediatric patients and their families. For these reasons, not only should SDOH integration be intentional, but also be ongoing and built from week to week to allow students time to reflect on the ways SDOH impact children and their families. Because SDOH does not occur within a vacuum, nor is it siloed, nursing students need opportunities outside of traditional textbook learning to apply skills of assessing and addressing SDOH in pediatric settings. Faculty must rise to the occasion to find and create these opportunities for students. However, faculty have many other competing demands that require their time and attention. Therefore, institutional support in the form of time and resources can greatly enhance faculty's ability to devote the time required to intentionally and frequently integrate SDOH.

Mental Health Nursing

Shaquita Starks

Background

The NHWSN SDOH framework is integral to understanding and examining how social factors such as culture, environment, social conditions, and policy impact the mental health outcomes of individuals across the life span. This framework was applied in a mental health course module for undergraduate nursing students to help them learn and identify SDOH associated with behavioral and mental health, and growth and development among Black, indigenous, and people of color (BIPOC) youth. The students learned about the following SDOH conditions that impact the behavioral and mental health outcomes of BIPOC youth: (a) lack of access to culturally sensitive and equitable mental healthcare, (b) community dynamics such as neighborhood policing, (c) lack of social support, (d) tradition, (e) identity, (f) religion and spirituality, and (g) the quality and conditions of schools, community environments, transportation, and housing. Students also learned about diagnostic disparities among BIPOC youth and broader implications for their behaviors. The students provided creative ways in which they would intervene with youth experiencing adversity and provided thoughtful feedback regarding culturally appropriate and sensitive art interventions.

Course Description

NRSG 411 *Mental Health Nursing* is a theory course that focuses on diverse concepts and principles merged from the sciences and humanities to the professional and specialized practice of psychiatric mental health nursing. This course examines comprehension and skills attainment to care for the mental health of patients across the continuum of care. This course is one out of five courses offered throughout Emory University involved in the Arts and Social Justice (ASJ) fellowship created by the Emory College Center for Creativity and Arts (CCA), and the Ethics and Arts program of the Emory University Center for Ethics. The program paired six Emory faculty with six Atlanta artists to collaborate and advance racial and social justice through their coursework. Students completed assignments and engaged with ASJ Fellows, Dr. Shaquita Starks (course coordinator) and Miranda Kyle, Arts & Culture program manager for the Atlanta Beltline, and other local Atlanta artists to learn about art activism, art interventions, and to gain an increased awareness and understanding of social inequities and diagnostic disparities in mental health among BIPOC youth. The course module included an overview of diagnostic criteria for conduct and impulse control disorders, a primer on adverse childhood experiences, and social determinants of health such as poverty, racial inequity, and discrimination.

A primary objective of this course and the associated art project was to help students develop strategies to collaborate with the community, parents, and school systems to bring awareness about the consequences of mental health disparities among BIPOC youth (e.g., mass incarceration and excessive policing). Course materials for this module included readings from the course textbook, the psychiatric diagnostic manual, nonfictional autobiographical readings, documentaries, lectures, evidence-based resources, and related peer-reviewed material. The overall goal of this course module was to empower students to facilitate change through awareness, art activism, and advocacy.

AACN Essentials Domain 1: Knowledge for Nursing Practice, Domain 2: Person-Centered Care, Domain 3: Population Health

Description of Course Assignment

The course opened with an overview of the pillars of the NHWSN SDOH framework and a discussion about factors such as poverty, racial inequity, discrimination, and racism. In addition to SDOH, intergenerational and historical trauma was highlighted, which heavily and more adversely impacts BIPOC youth. A transdiagnostic pedagogical approach was employed to teach students to conceptualize youth's symptomatology within the context of systems of oppression to de-pathologize BIPOC youth's presentation and to explicitly name more significant systemic problems rather than focusing on a reductionist diagnostic approach [10]. Students learned about multiple culturally relevant arts interventions and therapeutic community-level art (e.g., graffiti and mural painting) to engage and support youth experiencing mental distress and trauma.

Three assignments were created for students to complete. The first assignment included a 2-min recorded critical self-reflection detailing students' life stressors, traumatic events, or both. This assignment aimed to increase students' self-awareness of their experiences, resources, and supports. Students detailed their self-care engagement, creative stress coping strategies, adverse or traumatic life experiences, and how they learned their preferred type of creative self-care (i.e., learned from family, friends, or mental health professionals). The second assignment included three scenarios using existing audiovisual media with BIPOC youth ages six and older with behavior-related diagnoses and substance use issues. They were either arrested or victims of excessive force by school resource officers or police within their schools or neighborhood. Students selected one of three scenarios and identified the following:

1. SDOHs at play within the scenario.
2. Type of trauma impacting the youth.
3. Art intervention or therapy they would use with rationale for selecting (i.e., painting, drawing, and music).
4. Actions they would take to implement their chosen therapy to improve outcomes for the youth.

In this assignment, students were asked to describe source imagery for the muralist. From their descriptive narratives, a word cloud was created to determine the common themes among the students and provided to the muralist who transformed their words into a mural. The mural was painted by community members and students enrolled in the course with assistance from the muralist on the Atlanta Beltline, a former railway corridor now composed of green spaces and trails that circle the core of Atlanta, GA (see Fig. 5.2).

Fig. 5.2 Photo of students painting murals from their narratives

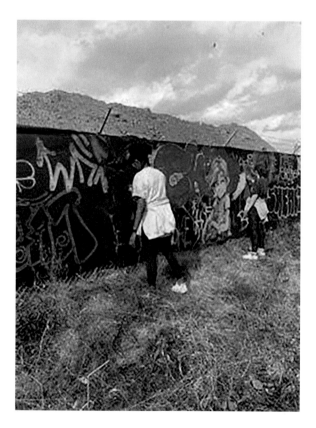

Student Assignment Exemplars

The last assignment included a reflection on the student's learning experience. Students were asked to address at least one of the following questions:

1. What stood out to you the most or surprised you completing this project?
2. What was the most interesting or important thing you learned through this course?
3. What important question(s) remain unanswered for you or not yet understood?
4. How will what you've learned from the Arts Social Justice assignments and readings impact how you serve BIPOC youth as a nurse in the future?

The following are selected student responses:

I loved learning about the intersection between arts and social justice and how this can improve the trajectory of individuals and overall health of a community. One question I have that remains unanswered is how to exactly integrate this content into my practice as a nurse. As nurses, specifically bedside, a large portion of our jobs is to administer medications and carry out treatments as ordered by the doctor. Of course, we practice therapeutic communication and building trusting relationships with patients as well. I understand that we could likely educate youth or parents of youth on the benefits of participating in art, but is there a more direct way we could introduce patients to art therapy at the bedside?

It was most impactful for me to read the stories and watch the videos that depicted how children have been impacted by SDOH that are out of their control, including the concept of the school-to-prison pipeline. It was surprising for me to watch the harmful experiences that many children endure, including violent force by authorities, as it is not something that I have experienced directly in my personal life.

In Part 2 of the assignment, the background information of each case stood out to me, as there were many underlying factors that contributed to the presentation of the scenarios. However, individuals are often wrongly accused or diagnosed due to the surface image of the specific situation, without including the SDOH in the perspective. As a nurse, I plan to serve BIPOC youth from an unbiased and compassionate perspective. It saddens me to see the experiences that many persevere through, yet they are often not considered to be uncommon. In my role on the healthcare team, I will be mindful of the hidden factors that may be contributing to the health presentation of a child within a situation. This may involve investigating their home life, social support networks, past trauma, as well as many other factors. By taking the time to engage with each individual, I may better support their unique needs and treat them holistically.

The concept of the school-to-prison pipeline was what surprised me most when completing this project. School is something that I grew up seeing as an opportunity and an institution that is there to serve its students. However, this "Arts & Social Justice" module showed me that this is not the reality for many students, especially those from disadvantaged backgrounds.

Based on these assignments, 29 students (76%) said they would change their practice and seek more information on the subject. Thirty-six students (92%) replied that their compassion for BIPOC youth experiencing adversity increased because of this assignment, and 31 students (79%) responded that their understanding of how SDOH influenced youths' mental health outcomes increased.

Reflection: Faculty

This assignment highlighted issues such as racism, health inequities and disparities, and poorer behavioral and mental health treatment which are long-standing and systematically reinforced issues impacting BIPOC youth in the United States. BIPOC youth are more likely to receive behavior-related diagnoses (e.g., disruptive, impulse control, and conduct disorder) than White youth. White youth are likely to receive diagnoses of neurodevelopmental and mood disorders (e.g., autism spectrum disorder, attention deficit hyperactivity disorder (ADHD), or adjustment disorder) [11].

Pharmacology for Nursing Practice

Kenneth Mueller and Christina Bhatia

Background

Historically, minimal SDOH discussions occurred within pharmacology courses at the Nell Hodgson Woodruff School of Nursing (NHWSN). Barriers to inclusion included time constraints and lack of knowledge. When SDOH discussions occurred, they primarily focused on medication access, cost, and affordability. However, with the development of the NHWSN SDOH Four Pillar Framework, the pharmacology course was restructured to allow for more appropriate inclusion of SDOH.

During the restructuring, pharmacology faculty spent extensive time identifying and researching SDOH topics that related to pharmacology. There are scant resources and information available on this topic, and faculty sought out resources such as conferences, podcasts, and recent publications. After identification of appropriate topics, faculty then established a framework to integrate these topics throughout the semester.

The first 2 weeks of the semester focused on developing foundational knowledge of pharmacology, including application of key principles such as pharmacokinetics and pharmacodynamics across the lifespan. During this foundational period, faculty also introduced the NHWSN SDOH Four Pillar Framework. The students were instructed that throughout the remainder of the semester they will learn pharmacology and the influences of SDOH within pharmacology and patient health.

Course Description

NRSG 508MN   This course provides students with an understanding of pharmacokinetics, pharmacodynamics, and pharmacogenomics when treating selected illnesses. Emphasis will be on nursing management of drug therapies in patients across the lifespan with application to the clinical setting.

AACN Essentials Domain 1: Knowledge for Nursing Practice

Examples of weekly pharmacology topics with associated SDOH foci are listed below.

	Pharmacology schedule	Examples of NHWSN SDOH pillars and topics
1	Pharmacology foundation: Pharmacokinetics, pharmacodynamics, pharmaceutics	Introduction of NHWSN SDOH Four Pillar framework
2	Pharmacology foundation 2: Lifespan considerations, medication safety and error reduction, principles of pharmacology	Social/Policy: Racism in medicine (use of race in eGFR) Environmental: Pharmacy deserts, climate change
4	Respiratory system (upper/lower): Asthma, COPD, allergies	Environmental: Exposure and asthma
5	Infectious diseases part 1: Antibiotics and vaccines	Policy/social: Racism in medicine (red man syndrome) Cultural/policy/social/environmental: Vaccine access, research, and hesitancy
6	Infectious diseases part 2: Antivirals, antifungals, antitubercular, antiprotozoal	Social/environmental: HIV prevalence rates COVID-19 treatment disparities
7	Hematology: Coagulation modifying agents, anemia	Policy/social: Clopidogrel (Hawaii Lawsuit)
10	Cardiology part 2: Heart failure, angina, dysrhythmias	Social/policy: Racism in medicine (First race based drug BiDil®)
11	Pain management: Opioids, NSAIDs, migraines, gout	Social/policy: War on drugs
13	Central nervous system part 2: Psychotherapeutics, anxiety/sleep, epilepsy	Social/policy: History of zolpidem and FDA drug approval

Description of Course Activities and Assignments

Pharmacology coursework includes weekly assignments, quizzes, and exams throughout the semester. Weekly assignments consist of *multiple choice* and *select all that apply* questions centered around the current weekly topic. These questions are written to evaluate student identification and understanding of drug classes and drug prototypes, and require students to identify common drug suffixes, indications, mechanisms, adverse effects, administration, cautions, contraindications, notable drug–drug or drug–food interactions, and other essential counselling points. Faculty incorporate SDOH *multiple choice* or *select all that apply* style questions periodically into weekly assignments to gauge student understanding of the SDOH topics.

One example SDOH lecture topic is racism in medicine. This SDOH topic is incorporated throughout multiple lectures including precision medicine and pharmacogenomics, pharmacokinetics and renal function, antibiotics, heart failure, and more. Faculty introduce examples of racism in medicine and describe how race has been used as a biological construct in patient treatment. Students then watch a TED Talk video titled, *The problem with race-based medicine by Dorothy Roberts*.

A specific lecture example of racism in medicine includes the use of race as a biological marker when estimating a glomerular filtration rate (eGFR). The use of race as a biological marker was found to cause inaccurate measures of renal function, which could lead to a vast array of consequences [12]. In 2021, the National Kidney Foundation (NKF) and the American Society of Nephrology (ASN) issued a report that all laboratories should remove the race modifier when using an equation to determine eGFR [13].

Another lecture example of racism in medicine is the FDA approval of the first "race-based drug," BiDil® for the treatment of heart failure in self-identified African Americans. Faculty remind students that race is a social construct, not a biological construct [14]. Faculty argue that approval of a "race-based drug" is misleading and inappropriately links race as a biological construct. This false assumption perpetuates racism in medicine.

Yet another example of racism in medicine is the use of the term *Red Man Syndrome* to identify a vancomycin flushing reaction. The term *Red Man Syndrome* has been used as a slur against Native Americans and Indigenous peoples, and trains healthcare professionals to identify these symptoms based only on the appearance of a Caucasian male [15]. Usage of this term continues racism in medicine and can lead to poor training and understanding of vancomycin's adverse effects and diagnosis. In 2021, a conglomerate of leading infectious disease groups including the Infectious Disease Society of America (IDSA), released a statement supporting the removal of the term *Red Man Syndrome* and replacing the term with *Vancomycin Infusion Reaction.*

Faculty also make it a point to discuss that while racism in medicine is a major SDOH theme, other vulnerable populations are also impacted by SDOH. An example that is used during lecture includes the history of zolpidem tartrate (Ambien®). Zolpidem tartrate was approved for use by the FDA in 1992. One year later, the NIH Revitalization Act of 1993 was passed, which directed the NIH to establish guidelines for the inclusion of women and minorities in clinical research [16]. Unfortunately, zolpidem tartrate was already out on the market. After years of post-marketing reports about women disproportionately experiencing adverse effects, the FDA recommended that women start on a lower dosage of zolpidem tartrate compared to men [17].

Student Assignment Exemplars

A sample question from a weekly assignment that is used to help evaluate student understanding of racism in medicine:

Select All That Apply: Which of the following are **biological** constructs/markers that can be used to identify appropriate drug dosing?

A. Race
B. **Sex**
C. **Bodyweight**
D. Socioeconomic status
E. Religion

Reflection: Faculty

During open discussions about SDOH conditions, student interaction was overwhelmingly positive. Students were appreciative of difficult conversations and inclusion of SDOH content into the curriculum. Students also contributed their own knowledge and experiences of SDOH conditions within medicine. Faculty end-of-semester surveys received high remarks about SDOH inclusion, and several student survey comments discussed that an appropriate amount of time was dedicated to SDOH in the pharmacology course, and that they appreciated the SON's initiative on SDOH inclusion. A minority of students felt like SDOH content felt out of context within a pharmacology course. One commented that the focus should be entirely on drug content, given the heavy science behind understanding drug mechanisms, adverse effects, contraindications, drug–drug interactions, and administration. A few students were resistant to sensitive topics such as racism in medicine and felt conflicted on select topics that may have been contradictory to their current beliefs or understanding.

One major challenge for faculty was time management. Prior to SDOH inclusion, time management was already a primary concern given that pharmacology is a three-credit hour course. With hundreds of drugs and drug classes to cover in one semester, faculty must find a balance of quality versus quantity in course content. Incorporating SDOH into a crammed course initially served as a major obstacle. However, faculty adjusted for this by identifying appropriate lecture topics, and then using brief, but frequent discussions of SDOH dispersed throughout the semester. Faculty also met with other instructors to review redundancy of SDOH content and pharmacology content (such as pharmacology content coverage in courses like Mental Health Nursing and Maternity and Reproductive Health).

Another challenge was the lack of faculty knowledge about SDOH content and difficult conversations. The SON developed faculty training modules on the NHWSN's SDOH Four Pillar Framework and assigned faculty to complete the SDOH training, which helped build foundational knowledge. Faculty felt that current pharmacology textbooks contain insufficient knowledge and resources for appropriate discussion of SDOH. Faculty then spent a large amount of independent time researching SDOH topics that could be appropriate for a pharmacology course. This included attending national conferences, listening to podcasts, reviewing published literature, and reading through any other available resources. Many SDOH topics that were identified are sensitive and possibly triggering to students, so faculty also spent time researching ways to approach difficult conversations in the classroom. Emory University's Center for Faculty Development and Excellence (CFDE) provided some teaching resources such as *Navigating Difficult Classroom Discussions* to help faculty prepare.

Art and Science of Nursing Practice

Lori A. Modly, Alyssa Meadows, Lindsey Allen, Isake Slaughter and Caitlyn Plattel

Background
Teaching a nurse to recognize the client through a lens of intersectionality is key to providing individualized patient care. To understand the client, the hospital, and the United States healthcare system, students must be taught the history, policies,

advantages, and barriers surrounding health and wellness. The concept of noncompliance is receding, and in its place is the nurse's ability to communicate with the patient and healthcare team to determine the barriers to wellness in a person's life. The SDOH are key pillars to unlocking factors contributing to patient and community health and wellness.

Course Description

NRSG 510 This course provides students with fundamental principles of nursing and clinical practice including an introduction to critical thinking, bioethics, nursing process, evidence-based practice, communication, health promotion/disease prevention, informatics, SDOH, and person- and family-centered care. This course is designed for our master's in nursing pre-licensure students. These students are second-degree students who are uniquely qualified to leverage their professional and life experience to further the profession of nursing.

This course is set up in three segments, the first covers an introduction to healthcare and the nursing profession, nursing scope of practice and ethics, SDOH, history of racism in medicine, and person-centered care. The second covers hospital policy and procedures, clinical judgment, the nursing process, interpersonal and therapeutic communication, quality, and safety. Finally, patient education, the wellness model, nursing theory, death and grieving, and resilience.

AACN Essential Domain 1: Knowledge for Nursing Practice, Domain 2: Person-Centered Care Domain 3: Population Health, Domain 6: Interprofessional Partnerships, Domain 7: Systems-Based Practice, Domain 9: Professionalism, Domain 10: Personal, Professional, and Leadership Development

Description of Course Assignment

The initial assignment is a student SDOH Book Club. Students choose from a curated list of book titles specifically addressing SDOH, and/or the human condition. These titles range from biographies, novels, historical fiction, and personal accounts. These are chosen from assorted topics, cultural perspectives, socioeconomic factors, racism, ableism, climate change, environmental health, ethics, and person-centered care. The student chooses a book to read and then creates an artistic representation of the book's theme. To facilitate student access to the books on the list, hyperlinks to the University Library or free access resources were included. A small grant was obtained to purchase a few physical copies of the books not available from one of the above resources. A request went out to faculty and staff for additional book donations, establishing a *SDOH Lending Library* for student use.

After reading the book the students complete a creative project to showcase the theme of their chosen title. The students' creative project can be presented in the form of an original painting, a sculpture, a photo, a song, or a 50-word mini-saga. Students can also choose to create digital artwork or make a photo collage. Students upload their artwork on a single slide onto an electronic discussion board. For the final portion of the project students substantively comment on two peer submissions within the electronic discussion board. Prompts for this post included, but were not limited to: "What about the artwork spoke to you? Can you discern the theme or message of the book from this piece of art? Does this piece motivate you to investigate more about the topic."

The creative aspect of this assessment is intentional in nature. I want the students to see these issues or barriers in healthcare and the ways in which individuals and communities deal with them in an art form. That the human condition is not just science and medical diagnosis. Students are encouraged to read their chosen book and reflect on the four pillars of the NHWSN SDOH Four Pillar Framework: social, environmental, cultural, and policy. How do the characters in the story benefit or suffer disadvantages within these pillars? Students are asked to reflect on how racism, ableism, and other forms of discrimination impact all aspects of a person's life. Treating a health condition is an evidence-based practice, however, navigating the barriers to individual wellness is an art form. The nursing process is key to our interactions with individuals seeking care, but often it is the art of the profession, therapeutic communication, problem solving, and coordinating care that makes the lasting impact.

This artistic exploration then leads directly into the larger learning assessment in the class; a scholarly paper describing an issue in professional nursing. The student is to build upon the theme they read about in the SDOH book. They will conduct a scholarly literature review to support their paper. They begin by describing the history and background of the issue. Next, they examine this issue's impact on professional nursing or healthcare. Lastly, the students use nursing, health or change theory to describe how they as individuals, the profession of nursing, or society can move this issue forward.

Student Assignment Exemplars

Book Presentation and Student Reflection by Alyssa Meadows (Fig. 5.3)

The book presentation assignment was a unique learning experience. With nursing school having such a heavy course load focusing on health and science concepts, it was nice to have an assignment focusing on social aspects impacting healthcare. I have always loved to read, but it can be so hard to find the time to read for pleasure in nursing school. I enjoyed having the opportunity to choose a topic to explore from a large selection of books. I wanted to make the most of the opportunity to read, and this assignment allowed me to slow down and take time to enjoy the experience of reading the book. Being given the choice of creating something to summarize the book's topic allowed me to explore more deeply what the book meant to me and gave me the freedom to be creative in a medium that I am comfortable with. I have always enjoyed writing freely and this gave me the opportunity to craft something meaningful to me. I think that having that creative outlet and freedom allowed me to learn more deeply as well. Because it was a topic I am interested in and that is personal to me, I was able to take it in a way that is different than if I had been assigned something that I might have had less interest in or if I had only had one

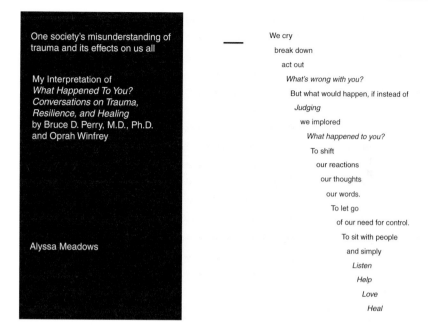

One society's misunderstanding of
trauma and its effects on us all

My Interpretation of
What Happened To You?
Conversations on Trauma,
Resilience, and Healing
by Bruce D. Perry, M.D., Ph.D.
and Oprah Winfrey

Alyssa Meadows

We cry
break down
act out
What's wrong with you?
But what would happen, if instead of
Judging
we implored
What happened to you?
To shift
our reactions
our thoughts
our words.
To let go
of our need for control.
To sit with people
and simply
Listen
Help
Love
Heal

Fig. 5.3 Book presentation: *What Happened to You? Conversations on Trauma, Resilience, and Healing* [18]

option of how to present. I also think it was great that we were able to see the topics that our fellow classmates explored and view their presentations. Many of the displays made me really feel the weight of the topics they chose and how different things impact people and their health. Overall, I think this assignment gave us an opportunity to see a more holistic view of healthcare by allowing us to use our unique experiences to create art that speaks to ourselves and others.

Book Presentation by Lindsey Allen (Fig. 5.4)

This book club assignment provided a deeper cultural context into various aspects of healthcare for me. Encouraging exploration of social determinants of health (SDOH) was personally appreciated because I gained a new understanding of an underserved population that I was ignorant toward. The book I chose was Fresh fruit, broken bodies: Migrant farmworkers in the United States. This may have just been a great book, or seven chapters of someone's life's work, however, it changed how I view the system that is such a disservice to migrant farmworkers in this country. It gave me a new appreciation for access to fresh fruits and vegetables, and a window to see what it costs these workers physically, mentally, and emotionally. It forced me to look beyond the news and opinions and step into their world, even if just for a minute. As humans there are stereotypes that often blind us to realities; however, as nurses, we must look beyond to foster an equitable system.

Fig. 5.4 Book
presentation: *Children of
the Land (picture created
by Connor Swan)* [19]

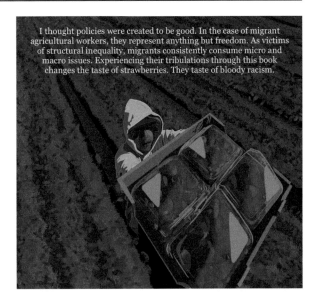

Fig. 5.5 Book
presentation: *I Know Why
the Caged Bird Sings* [20]

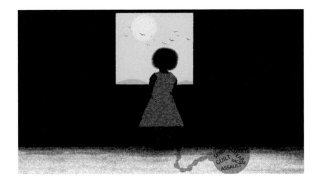

Book Presentation and Student Reflection by Isake Slaughter (Fig. 5.5)

For my SDOH book club assignment, I created digital artwork to showcase my artistic representation of the book *I Know Why the Caged Bird Sings* by Maya Angelou. Socioeconomics is a key theme presented throughout this book and a topic that I am very passionate about. Maya Angelou had experienced a great deal of tribulations and inequalities in her life which often made her and the people in her community feel trapped and helpless. In my visual, the bars and the ball and chain are symbolic of the physical, mental, social, and emotional restraints of life's injustices. However, through the window, she can still envision her hopes and dreams, and better days to come. This is the same ideology that I would like to carry with me throughout my nursing career. I found this assignment to be very engaging and thought provoking. It enabled me to be self-reflective on my own experiences and reality, while also gaining a new perspective.

Fig. 5.6 Book presentation: *Walk in My Combat Boots (picture created by Connor Swan)* [21]

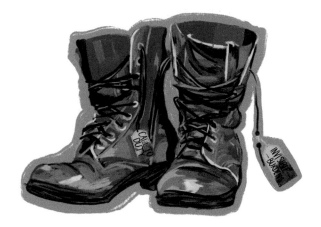

Book Presentation and Student Reflection by Caitlyn Plattel (Fig. 5.6)

Walk in My Combat Boots by James Patterson and Matt Eversmann is an extraordinary collection of memories and stories, from men and women who have proudly served our country. The SDOH Book Club discussion gave me the creative freedom to showcase what I felt was the underlying theme of the book: the invisible burdens that must be enlightened and educated upon to achieve veteran-specific trauma-informed care, within our healthcare systems. Seeing as there were an overwhelming number of different accounts of our military members' time in service, I found that it would be most impressionable and powerful to highlight the individual traumas that veterans carry each day but are often unknown to healthcare providers. Undoubtedly, this project left me empowered to strive to break the barriers that impede nursing practice and veteran healthcare.

Reflection: Faculty

Throughout this course the SDOH themes resurface in each lecture. Students oftentimes are the ones to point out the interconnectedness of SDOH and care. Taking the approach of allowing students to investigate their chosen issue in nursing/healthcare fostered a sense of curiosity. The students reported that they felt empowered by understanding specific examples of how SDOH innervates every aspect of individual or community care. They understand how to assess client needs and have the resources to find an evidence-based practice to meet those needs. During the second month of the course, faculty began reserving the last 10 min of class to discuss students' book choices, and the issues they were researching. Students were eager to have a safe space to share what they were learning, how they saw these issues expressed in their clinical environments, they also spoke with authority and enthusiasm regarding how to move this issue forward.

Social Responsibility and Bioethics

Rasheeta Chandler and Jessica Wells

Background

There is growing recognition of the negative impact of racism and bias and its disproportionate effect on health outcomes for Black communities, LGBTQAI+ communities, low-income, and rural communities. This growing recognition has led to an increase in accountability of healthcare professionals, specifically preparing nurses in health equity and social justice as part of the larger educational curriculum and training. In fact, the American Nurses Association (ANA) Code of Ethics compels nursing education to "firmly anchor students in nursing's professional responsibility to address unjust systems and structures, modeling the profession's commitment to social justice..." (p. 36) [22]. Whether at the bedside or within the community, the nurse should be prepared to amplify the profession's commitment to provide and advocate for high-quality and safe care for all patients in an array of settings. Nurses are often the first line of contact for the patient within the healthcare system and must assist the patient to navigate complex health, social, cultural, and even political aspects that impact their health and wellbeing. Nurses play a critical role as social justice advocates and must be prepared to recognize and address biases and ethical dilemmas that may impact the care and safety of their patients.

Course Description

NRSG 309 Social Responsibility and Bioethics in Nursing introduces a social responsibility framework as a model of professional nursing practice. The goal of the course is for students to develop essential skills to provide compassionate, patient-centered care and interpersonal skills to establish effective professional relationships. This course also offers an experiential learning component where the students obtain 20 service-learning hours during the semester. The goal of the didactic lectures is to engage first semester traditional BSN students in health equity and ethical concepts and to guide students to process new or difficult information through safe discussions and inflections. Course lessons cover topics on unconscious or implicit bias, social responsibility in nursing, anti-racism, cultural humility, and bioethics and ethical dilemmas in healthcare. Here, we present the course content that helped convey constructs of the NHWSN SDOH Four Pillar Framework [23].

AACN Essentials Domain 2: Person-Centered Care, Domain 9: Professionalism

Description of Course Assignment

A lecture focused on bioethics and ethical dilemmas in healthcare use a product from EthicsGame™ [24]. Students are navigated to complete Ethics Exercise™ that provides learners the opportunity to hone their knowledge of a typical nursing code of conduct. The exercises are based on multiple-choice questions that are designed to reinforce a professional code of conduct within the context of an ethical dilemma. Students complete exercises that covered two ethical dilemmas (1) fraudulent licensure and (2) incompetence/negligence. The fraudulent licensure exercises explore issues that may exceed the scope of nursing practice. The exercises hone a learner's knowledge of typical nursing code of conduct within the context of ethics. The learning objectives include avoiding and responding to issues of fraudulent licensure; identifying issues surrounding scope of practice; and exploring appropriate responses to Board of Nursing actions. The second ethical topic, incompetence, and negligence, explores issues of personal responsibility. This exercise explores factors that impact or impair a nurse's decision-making and the ability to provide safe patient care. The learning objectives for the incompetence and negligence exercises include effectively dealing with drug and alcohol use and abuse; avoiding incompetence due to personal illness or disability; and avoiding negligence and gross negligence.

After completion of the exercises, the class debriefs on the topics and their responses to the exercises. Many students reflect on how many of the ethical questions seem not to have a clear answer but to have more than one answer as the appropriate response to the dilemma. Students are assured that many dilemmas require critical thinking and critical reflection on the best answer or answer that will cause the least amount of harm for the patient. Ethical dilemmas in healthcare are not always black and white but often dwell in the gray area. Critical thinking and sound knowledge of the nurse's code of conduct are the foundation to help guide a nurse's judgment to ethical decision-making.

The Ethical Lens Inventory™ (ELI) [24] is employed to provoke decision-making based on students' values and perspectives. Students are asked to complete an assessment that probes 36 pairs of statements or words. More specifically, the assessment seeks to determine what values are most important to them or how they would act in certain situations. Once students complete the assessment, as a homework assignment, they receive a report that describes their preferred lens. We debrief in a class session, that aims to have students identify their fundamental ethical position per the ELI, so that they can better understand how to empathetically consider the social determinants that impact the lives of patients. In this lecture, the implications of SDOH that affect patients' ability to engage in and execute optimal health practices are central. Several SDOH-specific scenarios are revisited in class, students are polled to indicate their ethical positions, and open discussion ensues to realize diverse perspectives. The session concludes by having students reflect on the ELI activity and review the following:

- Agreement with their lens designations per ELI.
- Encouraging them to be mindful of their beliefs and consider the actions that might result.
- Because of that belief.
- Reminding them to be respectful of the values and commitments of others, like their patients.

Reflection: Faculty
Overall, feedbacks from student evaluations for this course were positive and applauded the course on "teaching us on issues that pertain to the current world (anonymous student)." This course discussed social topics that allowed for difficult but crucial conversations and exchange of thought-provoking dialogue. As nursing

faculty, it can be intimidating to teach hard social topics such as racism, biases, and social justice but feedback from the students help to affirm the need and acceptance of starting and leading these conversations for nursing students. It is imperative to establish the learning space as a safe space for these conversations. One student reflected in their evaluation "[the faculty member] is open to different viewpoints and I feel safe disclosing my personal opinions". A safe learning space allows nursing students to build their confidence as social change advocates and to later use their professional voices to advocate for social change and to advocate on behalf of their patients to promote health and wellbeing.

Nursing is an *art* and a science where art was amplified more in this course. As faculty, we must intentionally integrate the aspects of nursing that are not only anatomy and physiologically oriented, but consider the social, behavioral, and environmental (SDOH) aspects that impact patients' lives. The topics and approaches implemented in this course heightened students' ability to self-reflect, acknowledge their beliefs, but ultimately do what is best for patient health outcomes.

Evidence-Based Practice for the Professional Nurse

Wendy R. Gibbons, Erica Davis, and Harrison Diamond

Background

Evidence-Based Practice for the Professional Nurse can be a challenging course to teach with many hurdles to navigate. Master of Nursing (MN) students take this course in their second semester in nursing school, generally before they have experienced the breadth of the nursing role in individual, family, community, and population healthcare. Students can also view this as a "fluff" or "filler" course and not relevant to their future practice. Additionally, the students work in groups so they must also learn to navigate sometimes complex group dynamics to complete the work.

Previously, the course focused on utilizing evidence to support change in clinical practice. Since integrating the NHWSN SDOH Four Pillar Framework, the students' focus has shifted from exclusively clinically focused interventions to addressing the care culture, care inequities, and improving the health of communities. Since this shift, the students have demonstrated much more creativity and individuality in their EBP change projects. The students bring their backgrounds and life experiences to EBP and are learning that the culture of healthcare and care equity can be positively influenced by integrating these individual life experiences into their EBP projects.

Course Description

NRSG 542 Students will explore the research process and apply principles of evidence-based practice to clinical care delivery. Emphasis will be on search strategies and reviewing and synthesizing best research evidence for integration into practice.

AACN Essential Domain 1: Knowledge for Nursing Practice, Domain 4: Scholarship for Nursing Practice, Domain 5: Quality and Safety, Domain 8: Information and Healthcare Technologies

Description of Course Assignment

Students are asked to design a project highlighting an EBP change they developed through the critical appraisal of evidence on several topics ranging from alcohol treatment to pain management. The objective for this assignment involves students defining and assessing the influences of SDOH (cultural, social, environmental, and policy), on illness and wellness in nursing at the individual, family, community, and societal levels. The project is a culmination of several assignments throughout the semester where students are guided in the evaluation of patient populations and nursing populations in relation to their social contexts. Students construct a poster and written summary before giving a comprehensive presentation of the EBP change. They are asked how their findings are related to SDOH and what can be done in practice to ensure these areas of care are properly addressed. Faculty guide students' thought processes on caring for individuals and populations of interest in the areas of social, policy, cultural, and environmental aspects of health.

Student Assignment Exemplars (Figs. 5.7, 5.8, 5.9, 5.10, and 5.11)

Reflection: Faculty

One of the assignments the students completed was a project synthesis of their EBP literature research. It was a three-page summary of the multiple worksheets completed that were designed to develop a clinically relevant research question to address areas of nursing practice in need of improvement. Students were asked to address barriers to change and community stakeholders that might influence their intervention and targeted population. The process of identifying barriers to change and making adequate changes for EBP led to expanded conversations about the social aspects of care that need to be addressed for individuals who are to benefit from the standard of practice achieved through the EBP. Subsequently, students created a poster as a final product which they presented in class and further discussed their goals in attaining excellence by addressing the SDOH with their EBP project for their chosen populations.

Students verbalized understanding the importance of the context of care for individuals, families, and the larger community. Students were able to grasp the concepts of care coordination and resource management when caring for diverse groups and populations in the context of the social, environmental, political, and cultural aspects of care after completing this assignment. There were three key takeaways: (1) students were able to view the need for social aspects of care in different populations they explored, (2) students developed a clear direction for identifying the various aspects of care involved with the SDOH, and (3) students were able to identify barriers related to SDOH and therefore potential solutions for change to enhance healthcare interventions in nursing.

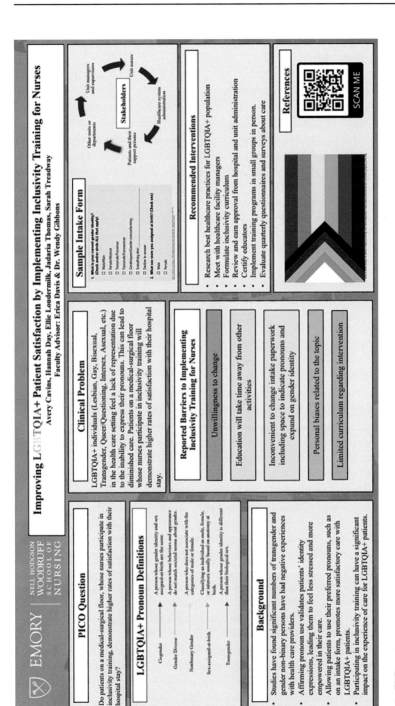

Fig. 5.7 EBP poster

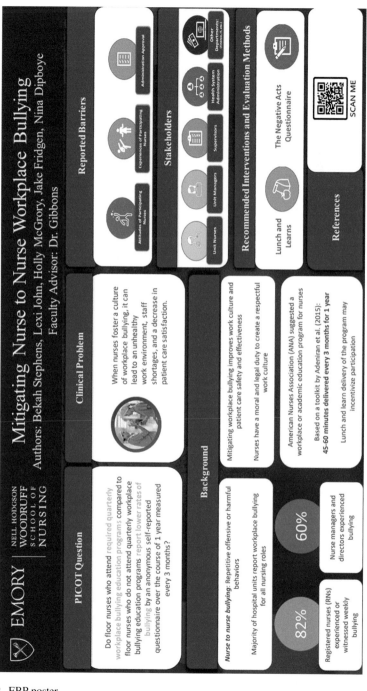

Fig. 5.8 EBP poster

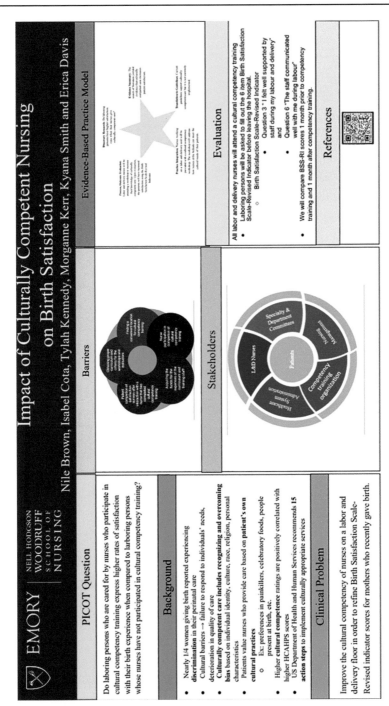

Fig. 5.9 EBP poster

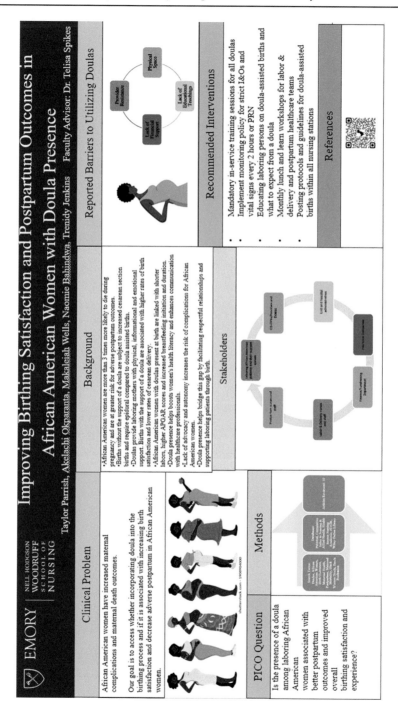

Fig. 5.10 EBP poster

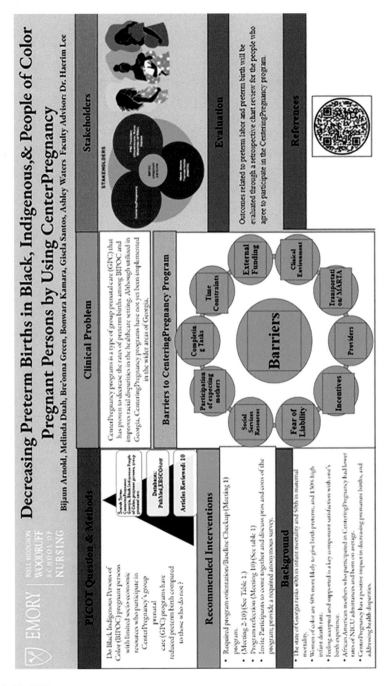

Fig. 5.11 EBP poster

Reflection: Student

Before this class, I only looked at SDOH within population health and health promotion realms. But now I know the possibilities for its use are limitless. Before the EBP class, I never realized how SDOH could be used as a tool to make interventions better or to appraise scholarly research to ensure you are using the best evidence possible. There are applications of SDOH that can be used in every setting and at every step in the nursing process and I look forward to utilizing SDOH in my practice as a nurse.

The first step of the nursing process is assessment. We often think about assessment in terms of doing the physical assessment and taking a comprehensive health history, but I believe adding in the SDOH as an assessment tool can be incredibly useful. Knowing how SDOH uniquely affects an individual can help better provide person-centered care during the course of treatment from admission to discharge. An aspect of SDOH I have seen a pattern emerge has been within the cultural aspect. While in the clinical setting, I see almost an apprehension or embarrassment of black women to ask for pain medications. A refrain I have heard repeatedly has been, "I'm not a junkie". I have to believe these women have had bad experiences in healthcare or the providers have not believed them when they were in pain in the past. I will make sure going forward that when I am discussing plan of care with individuals to stress pain management is an important goal we should work on together and that there are tools available to help meet those goals, including pharmacological. It is my goal that by normalizing this, patients will not feel apprehensive about asking for something they need.

Undergraduate Nursing Honors Program

Caroline Kee and Nicholas A. Giordano

Background

The delivery of safe high-quality care depends on the effective implementation and sustained evaluation of evidence-based practices by nurses practicing across care settings. However, to effectively do so, nurses of all licensures must be adequately prepared to interpret clinical research findings and, if needed, engage in the conduct of research. Therefore, nurse scientists in academic settings are well positioned to not only support nursing students cultivate an interest in research but also to assist them in understanding how to systematically assess the impact social determinants of health have on care outcomes across diverse patient populations utilizing systematic research approaches. This exemplar outlines one longitudinal assignment that achieves the dual objectives of engaging future nurses to develop the skills needed to interpret and engage in clinical research while simultaneously systematically examining differences in clinical outcomes based on social determinants of health.

Course Description

The Honors Program at NHWSN provides a challenging academic experience for the most intellectually gifted, motivated, and inquisitive BSN students. Students in the Honors Program explore issues that are relevant to nursing and society at an in-depth level. Honors Program participants build a dynamic network through cohort and mentoring methods of inquiry. Throughout their experience, Honors students have opportunities to develop skills related to the School of Nursing's core values: excellence, collaboration, social responsibility, innovation, and leadership. Honors students conduct research or a scholarly project, write a thesis and present their work. Honors students complete a series of four courses that prepare and support them to conduct an exemplary thesis project. Each semester the student works with a faculty mentor on iterative components of the thesis (e.g., refining the research question, reviewing the literature, outlining methods used, data collection, conducting data analyses, and synthesizing results). The resulting product from this coursework is an abstract submitted to an academic research conference. Collectively, these courses and their cumulative assignment work align with the American Association of Colleges of Nursing's Essentials for nursing education [1].

AACN Essentials Domain 1: Knowledge for Nursing Practice

Description of Course Assignment

The longitudinal nature of this assignment affords a unique opportunity to forge the next generation of BSN-prepared nurses who are prepared to prioritize research in their daily practice. After enrolling in the course, students are introduced to faculty and their research over a series of meet and greets in the first 2 weeks of the class. Faculty provide 10–15 min introduction of their research interests to the students and potential projects students can engage in over the course of four semesters. Next, students initiate coffee talks with faculty that align with their interests to discuss in detail what research project involvement would look like. Faculty identify students that they prefer to work with throughout the multipart course and agree to meet regularly to review student progress (e.g., every other week for 30 min). Each week students meet with their course faculty and classmates to gain foundational knowledge on research methods in tandem to applied research experience with faculty mentors.

Any research-based assignment can actively aid future clinicians to better recognize the root causes that affect both individual and population health. Specifically, this course-related assignment aligns with enabling students to explore the contributions of social factors and policies that contribute to health and wellness among patient populations that have historically been systematically marginalized from receiving evidenced-based pain management [25, 26]. Exploring how patients' relationships and interactions with health systems, specifically the clinicians within them, may impact health outcomes provides students with a data-driven approach to identifying systemic challenges faced by patients before entering clinical practice themselves and risk perpetuating similar biases. For example, in the assignment below the student examines through data potential differences in pain management provided to patients living with substance use disorders by race. These social factors can also be influenced by policies within the health system, such as limiting the amount of opioid medication dispensed based on pain scores. When paired with under assessment of pain, specifically among Black and African American patient populations, this may result in the misapplication of policies that systemically reduce the pain medication dispensed to alleviate pain in acute care settings compared to among non-Hispanic white patients [27]. Importantly, findings that these disparities persist can help inform the future implementation of multidimensional pain assessment, which focuses on pain's impact on functioning rather than intensity scores alone [28]. This assignment provides an exemplar of how to utilize data to help students identify how social determinants of health impact clinical care and subsequently patient outcomes, in the context of pain management.

Student Assignment Exemplar

Below is one example of a student assignment that demonstrates the student's emerging expertise in conducting research with a focus on SDOH. In this situation, a student had expressed interest in gaining experience conducting research with individuals diagnosed with substance use disorder and understanding how care needs differ in this patient population across segmented demographic presentations. At the time, the faculty mentor was leading a retrospective study using a large health record data repository examining demographic and clinical presentations among patients readmitted within 90 days after undergoing surgery due to an orthopedic injury. The student worked with the faculty member to leverage this data source to identify a subsample of individuals who were injured and had a co-occurring substance use disorder diagnosis. The student was able to successfully identify a subsample and examine differences in pain management treatment between patients with substance use disorder who identified as Black compared to those who identified as white. A summary of this mentored research investigation can be found below:

Background: On average, each year 8.9 million opioid prescriptions are dispensed to 3.9 million patients in the United States. Despite this volume of opioids prescribed, there is a disproportionate distribution and access to opioids across patients of different races and ethnicities. The average dose of prescription opioids was 36% lower among patients who identified as Black than white patients according to Medicare claims from 2016 to 2017. These differences are due to the explicit and implicit bias of clinicians and the incorrect belief that Black patient populations feel less pain than White patient populations. Yet, pain levels do not significantly differ between patients who are Black and patients who are white. Nine percent of the United States population lives with a substance use disorder (SUD). Overall, patients with substance use disorder often report increased pain scores, lengthy hospital stays due to pain, and slower pain resolution. Considering the increased pain management needs of patients with substance use disorder and the mistrust often reported among patients and their interactions with clinicians, pain may be inadequately managed in patients most affected by it.

Objective: This retrospective study aimed to identify the compounding influences of race and substance use disorder in prescription opioid doses to patients with orthopedic injuries seen at one of the largest level 1 trauma centers in the nation from. Specifically, this work compared the doses of prescribed opioids following orthopedic trauma between patients with substance use disorder who identified as Black or African American compared to patients with substance use disorder who identified as white.

Methods: This study utilized health record data from 1410 patients seen at a level 1 trauma center between 2018 and 2020 presenting with orthopedic injuries. Demographic and clinical characteristics, including average pain scores, were collected from the health records. All opioid medication utilized during hospitalization and received at discharged were tabulated and transposed as morphine milligram equivalents (MME). Separate multivariable generalized linear models were constructed to compare opioid medication dosage during hospitalization and at discharge between Black and white patients while adjusting for age, sex, injury severity, surgery, length of stay, and comorbidities.

Results: In progress.

Conclusions: In all healthcare systems, nurses are patient advocates. Due to the subjectivity of pain, it can be difficult to adequately manage pain without the use of nurse-led pain assessments. As patient advocates, nurses have the duty to strive for effective pain management for all of their patients by leveraging data from their routine pain assessments to inform the delivery of evidence-based optimal pain management from prescribers. With this research, we can develop tailored, clinician-focused education to reduce potential biases in prescribing to Black and White patients with SUDs presenting with orthopedic trauma. As nurses, we can recognize the likely bias among prescribers for our patients and work to ensure they do not affect pain management. By first illuminating existing differences in access to prescriptions across patients of various races, with and without substance use, we can help inform future nurse-led efforts, such as routine and unbiased pain assessments. These efforts can inform interventions and policies capable of narrowing health disparities.

Reflection: Faculty

Working with the student on this assignment enabled the faculty member to learn from the student on best approaches for mentoring emerging scholars, advance his program of research while simultaneously incorporating a new line of inquiry centered on characterizing disparities in pain treatment based on individuals living with substance use disorders. For example, in the conduct of this work the faculty member was able to receive feedback from the student on the best structure and frequency for meetings as well as how best to help the student form foundational knowledge on this subject area. This included designing, in partnership with the student, a monthly journal club to review and discuss articles on racially influenced disparities in pain assessment and management, pathophysiology of opioid-induced hyperalgesia, and stigma toward individuals living with substance use disorders. This work also helped the faculty member to illustrate the need for targeted clinical-level interventions to enable nurses to better assess pain among individuals with substance use disorders, across races, presenting in emergency department settings so as to inform the delivery of optimal multimodal pain management. This student-initiated effort also served as an opportunity to engage and collaborate with other senior investigators with dedicated programs of research centered on health disparities. This assignment is replicable to other faculty conducting research at academic health centers or community practice facilities with access to electronic health records. Faculty at other institutions can consider designing partnerships with faculty, clinician scientists embedded in health systems who are often already conducting research and quality improvement work, and students to advance emerging scholars' understanding of health disparities.

Advanced-Level Nursing Education Exemplars

Advanced Health Assessment

Amy Becklenberg, Elizabeth Downes, Autherine Abiri, and Maria-Bernarda Saavedra

Background

Advanced Practice Registered Nurses (APRNs) are in an ideal position to assess and address the social determinants of health (SDOH). Many APRNs work in communities in primary care settings, including federally qualified health centers, school-based health centers, and nurse managed centers. In these settings, APRNs are often in close proximity to where people "are born, live, learn, work, play and worship" [29]. In addition, APRNs can build trusting relationships with individuals and their families, with frequent encounters over many years. Equipping APRNs with the skills of assessing and addressing SDOH is essential for mitigating health disparities. The Advanced Health Assessment course is an ideal time for APRN students learning to incorporate assessing and addressing SDOH during every encounter.

Course Description

NRSG 544 Students enrolled in Advanced Health Assessment have a didactic lecture each week that focuses on one body system. For example, the first body system assessment discusses assessment of the Head, Eyes, Ears, Nose, and Throat (HEENT). The next week's lecture covers assessment of the neurologic system. The following week, assessment of the musculoskeletal system is the focus until assessment of all body systems has been taught.

AACN Essentials Domain 2: Person-Centered Care

Description of Course Assignment

Weekly SOAP Note Assignment As part of the Health Assessment Lab requirements, students are required to document their findings in the form of a Subjective, Objective, Assessment, and Plan (SOAP) note. Weekly lab scenarios are written at the problem focused level and students are required to address the following items for their SOAP Note Assignment each week (SDOH Framework Social Pillar).

The social pillar of the NHWSN SDOH Framework is addressed in each SOAP Note assignment submission. While the social history that students are required to gather from their "patient" in lab each week is not extensive, it reinforces the importance of assessing social determinants such as housing, social support, and employment, which may also provide insights into the individual's level of education, financial resources, language and health literacy and access to healthcare.

APRN students are taught that gathering a social history is required even for a simple episodic visit for a complaint such as headache or allergic rhinitis. When students are required to include a social history each time they document a visit, it reinforces the importance of social conditions when providing effective care.

Future opportunities for incorporating a more extensive assessment of SDOH could include enhancing the prompts within the social history for the environmental pillar, assessing the individual's community environment including green space, bike lanes, sidewalks, access to health foods, air pollution, access to healthcare settings, and involvement in faith-based institutions could all be incorporated into the social history section of the SOAP note template.

Student Assignment Exemplars

In the first example, the scenario included a 25-year-old female complaining of an earache for the past 3 days. The student included the following social history in her documentation:

Social History (SHx) Patient is a full-time graduate student obtaining her master's in public health and currently lives with two roommates in a three-bed and three-bath apartment. The patient does not smoke, consume alcohol, or does any illicit/recreational drugs. The patient notes that she copes with school stress by staying active, a combination of cardio and strength training 5–6 days a week. Patient notes she likes to cook and eats healthy. She usually likes to have oatmeal in the morning with fruit and a cup of decaffeinated coffee. For lunch she will eat grilled chicken salad. For dinner, she likes to have the same grilled chicken with broccoli rice and beans. Patient drinks a minimum of 2 liters of water every day. Patient notes she is sexually active, and her partner always uses a condom. Patient gets an average of 8 h of sleep every night. Patient states she has an adequate support system at school, home, and from her immediate family.

In the second example, the scenario included a 45-year-old male complaining of headaches for 2 days. The student included the following social history in her documentation:

Social History (SHx) Patient has worked at a car shop as a mechanic for the past 10 years. Recently divorced, lives alone in a one-bed one-bath apartment. Smokes one pack of cigarettes a day for the past 20 years. Drinks two beers every evening during the week and more than two beers on weekends. Denies recreational drugs.

Reflection: Faculty

The NHWSN SDOH four-pillar framework is the ideal model for nursing faculty to use when considering further integration of the SDOH into their teaching within the Advanced Health Assessment course for enhancing the didactic and lab content. Updates to the didactic content could include using the NHWSN SDOH four pillar framework during the first lecture of the semester *Health History and Interview Process* lecture. One PowerPoint slide could cover each of the four pillars and the lecturer could discuss how each pillar could relate to patient health. In addition, students could be required to address the four pillars within their SOAP note assignment each week in lab.

A more robust integration of the NHWSN SDOH four pillar framework into the Advanced Health Assessment course for APRN students better prepares APRN students to assess and address SDOH during each encounter. The Advanced Health Assessment weekly lectures and lab provide a unique opportunity for deeply embedding the importance of an SDOH mindset in our future APRNs. This approach will prepare APRNs to confidently embrace their role in forming more supportive relationships with individuals. It will also help them connect individuals to critically important resources within their community, thereby facilitating improvement of health outcomes and minimizing health disparities.

Omics in Health and Disease (PhD Course)

Irene Yang and Stephanie Lee

Background

Recognizing that health and disease are shaped by multiple, co-occurring, and multi-level domains of influence including biological and SDOH with impacts at levels ranging from the individual to larger society [30], this course strives to expose nurse researchers to the scientific and clinical possibilities of -omics research methods while incorporating a SDOH research lens [31]. Emphasizing a SDOH research lens helps students learn to ensure rigor of study design and prioritize outcomes that are contextualized to have the greatest impact on human health.

Course Description

The course provides a broad overview of various -omic fields of study including genomics, epigenomics, metabolomics, lipidomics, and microbiomics. The biology and theoretical principles underlying these methods are presented along with their application to knowledge discovery, precision medicine/nursing, and the development of targeted interventions to improve health outcomes. The collection of specimens, processing of samples, and lab analysis relevant to respective -omics methods are also reviewed. Practical, statistical, and ethical challenges related to research design and the gathering and interpretation of big data generated in studies employing these methods are also discussed. Through this course, students explore the possibility of incorporating one or more -omics methods into their own programs of research and evaluate and apply evidence-based knowledge about influences of social determinants (cultural, social, environmental, and political) on illness and wellness as they relate to -omics research.

AACN Essentials Domain 1: Knowledge for Nursing Practice, 2: Person-Centered Care

Description of Course Assignment

Throughout the course, students read multiple articles that serve as exemplars of -omic methods used in health research studies. Students are required to provide a one-page written critique of these articles using the guidelines below. As can be seen, students are asked to critically reflect on the study using an SDOH research lens. Of special interest is responding to the question—How does this research study address one or more social determinants of health (see Emory SON's Social Determinants of Health Framework) and/or have an impact on health equity? OR How could this study have been designed to better address a social determinant of health or have an impact on health equity?

Student Assignment Exemplar

Critique of Kris, M. G., Johnson, B. E., Berry, L. D., Kwiatkowski, D. J., Iafrate, A. J., Wistuba, I. I., Varella-Garcia, M., Franklin, W. A., Aronson, S. L., Su, P. F., Shyr, Y., Camidge, D. R., Sequist, L. V., Glisson, B. S., Khuri, F. R., Garon, E. B., Pao, W., Rudin, C., Schiller, J., Haura, E. B., … Bunn, P. A. (2014). Using multiplexed assays of oncogenic drivers in lung cancers to select targeted drugs. JAMA, 311(19), 1998–2006. https://doi.org/10.1001/jama.2014.3741 [32].

The primary objective of this study was to determine the frequency of ten oncogenic drivers (genomic alterations that impact cancer development and maintenance) in patients with lung adenocarcinomas. The secondary objectives were to define the co-occurrence of the drivers in a single tumor, use the data to select targeted treatments, and measure survival. Participants included in the study were required to have a stage IV or recurrent lung adenocarcinoma diagnosis with a Southwest Oncology Group (SWOG) performance status between 0 and 2 (0 meaning asymptomatic, 1 meaning symptomatic but fully ambulatory, and 2 meaning symptomatic but in bed less than 50% of the day). In addition to evaluating the study's purpose, methods, and analysis approach, this critique evaluates the article through a social determinants of health (SDOH) lens. Unfortunately, this study essentially ignores any considerations about SDOH, particularly with regard to the social and environmental conditions that influence health. In my opinion, this is a significant limitation. First, the authors fail to consider the influence of SDOH on the genomic milieu of a tumor. Environmental exposures, for example, may drive genetic alterations underlying cancer development yet environmental exposure factors considered in this study were limited to smoking history. The study did not consider critical exposures like secondhand smoke or occupational exposures like coal mining.

Second, the failure to consider social conditions in the design of this study severely limits the generalizability of study findings. Factors like racism, ethnicity, financial status, education, and occupation were not discussed. Financial status and education are two important factors that influence how a patient might approach cancer screening and treatment. Lack of health insurance or low health literacy present barriers to care making it unlikely for some to have been eligible to participate in this study. For this study, participants were only recruited from large academic medical centers, excluding anyone who did not receive cancer treatment at a large academic medical center. Rural populations often experience barriers to care due to distance from medical centers. The study could have recruited participants from smaller community hospitals in different parts of the country to see how and if oncogenic drivers differ in populations that might not have access to large academic medical centers. By ignoring SDOH factors, the authors fail to account for potential confounding factors that could be relevant, and they ignore ethical concerns about access to care and to clinical trials. This critique highlights the importance of SDOH considerations in the design and interpretation of clinical research.

Reflection: Faculty

This exemplar represents one example of how an SDOH lens was incorporated into the curriculum. A key objective of the course was for students to be able to effectively critique -omics research studies using an SDOH lens. This was the first journal critique of the semester and the featured student received encouraging comments for her ability to critique the study clearly, and thoughtfully in terms of its design, SDOH considerations, and conclusions.

The instrumental value and technological novelty of -omics methods frequently lend itself to studies focused on physiologic mechanisms without the context of broader SDOH. This course encourages intentional reflection on the intersection of -omics research and SDOH, preparing students to not only effectively critique -omics-related literature, but also to think through how studies utilizing -omics methods can be designed to elucidate biological mechanisms underlying the association between SDOH and disparate outcomes.

Reflection: Student

Throughout my entire PhD program, the values of health equity and equality have been woven into every class and prioritized as a crucial component of my education. Yet I was surprised to have these concepts as a focus of my -omics course, which to me is more "bench science" focused than other nursing courses. This course helped me learn to critically evaluate research articles with clear guidelines, and I appreciated how intentional course instructors were about asking students to critically evaluate and find the intersection of -omics techniques and SDOH. Not only did I learn new -omics-related vocabulary and methods, but my thinking also expanded to see the connection between the two and how -omics research can be designed to answer and explain biological or physiological mechanisms that contribute to health disparities. This course represents the best part about nursing research: its ability to negotiate the intersection of many different areas of science in a way that sets the foundation for creating evidence-based nursing practice, promoting equitable treatment of all people, and producing optimal patient outcomes.

Analysis of Complex Systems for Populations and Organizations (DNP Course)

Susan L. Swanson and Rebekah Elting

Background

Healthcare is challenged by complex interrelationships and difficult problems, including SDOH inequalities such as food, financial and housing insecurity, education, structural conflict, and access to affordable and equitable healthcare. Advanced practice nurses and those at the frontlines of healthcare are in a pivotal position to assess for SDOH and positively address factors contributing to patient and population health disparities and inequities. Systems thinking offers a holistic approach to complex problem solving directed toward transformative and sustainable change for individuals, populations, and organizations.

Course Description

NRSG 712 Analysis of Complex Systems for Populations and Organizations exposes students to complexity theory and systems thinking with a special focus on addressing issues in healthcare organizations and vulnerable populations. Students holistically evaluate a variety of problems by examining the interactions between parts of a system and how their emergent behaviors produce often unpredictable results in dynamic settings. By looking for the simple rules that underly all complex adaptive systems, learners will be able to frame and present strategies to transform care in a variety of domains (micro, meso, and macro), including those factors influencing SDOH, such as economic, social, educational, geographic, and structural challenges. By the end of the course, students should be better positioned to systemically identify and approach problems and solutions within their own organizations, projects, and course case studies, with more creativity, adaptability, and clarity for the implications of SDOH among vulnerable populations.

AACN Essentials Domain 7: Systems-Based Practice

Description of Course Assignment

This final assignment is asking you, as a systems thinker, to build upon, translate, and synthesize what you have learned in this course in a 7–10 min Zoom poster presentation. The poster should reflect the culmination of the work you have done, and feedback received from prior assignments and relevantly incorporate SDOH implications. For those unfamiliar with the value of a poster presentation, this is one of the most common ways you will communicate your work in an academic setting. A good poster makes a quick visual impression of the main takeaways of your work. It allows you to gain interest from others in your work and to network with like-minded or similarly positioned professionals who may help you promote your story and/or influence your work/practice/specialty. Please adhere to the following guidelines:

The poster sections in the template are categorically structured to assure you address the required elements for this assignment, which include:

- Statement of the problem
- Introduction
- Background
- Archetype
- Causal loop diagram
- Theoretical framework
- Discussion and recommendations
- Conclusion
- References

Students are welcome to alter the poster format based on the needs of their own work and their own creative approach. While your narrative is important, the key takeaways should be briefly presented in each section so that an uninformed observer is able to garner key points and easily interpret the issue, significance, opportunities, etc.

Student Assignment Exemplar (Fig. 5.12)

Reflection: Faculty

While many advanced practice nurses recognize they work within systems of care, having students evaluate contributing causes to the fatal medication error in a case study assignment, helped the instructor determine their level of systems and SDOH knowledge and complex problem-solving skills, early in the course. This group assignment set the stage for the scaffolding of follow-on assignments that incorporated SDOH and the students' problem area of interest. The early opportunities to analyze their own "wicked problems" (with consideration for SDOH), made students feel more engaged in applying the systems constructs learned in the course. In addition, students enjoyed two synchronous sessions with guest speakers discussing their systems approach to wicked problems in their hospital system and in another global community. These real-world examples enabled students to hear about transformative change in highly complex systems that came about by using the principles and tools they were learning in the course. The final poster presentation by the students and their peers served as an affirmation of their enhanced systems thinking knowledge and competencies. Incorporating complexity science and systems thinking as part of the core DNP curriculum, faculty are in a pivotal position to help advanced

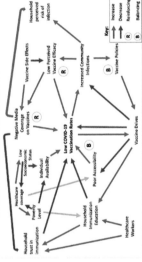

Fig. 5.12 Student poster presentation

practice nurses and those students on the front lines of healthcare, assess for SDOH and implement evidence-based approaches that constructively address factors contributing to the health disparities and inequities affecting patient and population health outcomes.

DNP Scholarly Project

Melissa A. Poole-DubinPhyllis Wright, and Jill B. Hamilton

Background
Through a scholarly project focused on meeting the AACN Essentials (2021), as well as integration of SDOH, the student pursued important indicators that affect populations and began molding the focus for future practice. The multi-semester DNP project builds upon the semester before, develops tools for scholarly work, dissemination of information, and promotes healthcare transformation for the practice students to enter post-graduation.

Course Description
NRSG 715, 716, 717, 721   The Doctor of Nursing Program at NHWSN provides a stepwise approach to guide students through their chosen scholarly project across four semesters. Students begin with identifying a purpose for the project by building a foundation through scholarly literature search and appraisal, analyzing system-driving factors, and linking these factors to a theory or framework. The second semester continues with project development guided by the SDOH. Students establish a site-specific project plan while collaborating with a sponsoring clinical/community partner and supported by a faculty mentor. Semester three continues with project implementation and a continued focus on SDOH. Project findings describe how effective the intervention is with alleviation of the problem and the influence of SDOH on the population addressed.

Description of Course Assignment
The DNP student's project applied evidence and evaluated the influences of SDOH on health outcomes. The NHW SDOH Four Pillar Framework provided a lens that examined the social, cultural, environmental, and policy conditions that impact the overall health at the individual and community levels, and whether these impact outcomes positively or negatively [23]. Including these conditions opens the opportunity to reach across familiar SDOH conditions and create a new understanding beyond archetypal conditions encountered and addressed in real-world nursing experience. The SDOH lens broadens the student's consideration of health challenges and outcomes when considering project goals as well as future practice initiatives. Instead of a common focus on physical aspects that create health opportunities or disparities, this project considered intangible contexts during project development, implementation, and evaluation. This foundation in SDOH leads to transforming healthcare to reach individual and population-level healthcare opportunities, access, and equity.

AACN Essential Domain 2: Person-Centered Care, Domain 4: Scholarship for Nursing Practice, Domain 7: Systems-Based Practice

Student Assignment Exemplar

The DNP project explored the perceptions of hospital-based social support among African American women with breast cancer. A secondary analysis of previously collected open-ended interviews guided this exploration of perceptions of social support groups among African American women with breast cancer. These interviews also provided insight into the low participation rates of hospital support group participation among these women. This qualitative analysis gave voice to the experiences of African American women with breast cancer. The experiences of these women also informed the larger body of quantitatively generated evidence that reports low numbers of African American women in hospital-based cancer social support groups.

Aim To better understand the perceptions African American women diagnosed with breast cancer have for hospital-based support groups and if those perceptions dissuade participation in these groups.

Design A qualitative descriptive design including criterion sampling, open-ended semi-structured interviews, and qualitative content analysis was used to guide this exploration.

Methods A qualitative descriptive design including criterion sampling, open-ended semi-structured interviews conducted between 2013 and 2020, and qualitative content analysis was used to guide this exploration.

Results Four themes related to perceptions of support groups emerged which included (a) social support from naturally occurring social networks, (b) the type of support from naturally occurring networks, (c) hospital-based support groups perceived as negative and lacking optimism, and (d) community-based support groups perceived as grounded in spirituality and humor.

Conclusion These breast cancer survivors perceived that hospital-based support groups were symptoms-based, focusing on grief, pain, and discontent around cancer which they perceived as negative experiences. In comparison, perceptions of African American community-based support groups were perceived as positive, spiritually grounded, finding purpose in the experience, and humor.

Impact Tailoring hospital-based support groups for underserved populations takes a holistic person, community, and culturally focused approach, benefiting not only the physical component but also the emotional, mental, and spiritual aspects of survivorship. African American breast cancer survivors in these interviews highlight the impact of community partnerships on individual health outcomes.

Reflection: Faculty

I have been principal investigator and led a series of studies to better understand the social and cultural conditions that influence health outcomes among African American cancer survivors. These studies have generally focused on the ways in which African Americans rely on support from family, friends, and their faith in God to persevere the struggles during life-threatening illnesses. My experience to date with nursing graduate students has generally been with PhD students, however, it was an absolute delight to work with Melissa on this DNP project.

I was introduced to Melissa through a faculty colleague who had a student interested in incorporating SDOH into a DNP project. Melissa expressed to me at our initial meeting of her interest in exploring the relevance of hospital support groups for African American women with breast cancer. I remembered hearing comments from the women I had interviewed in a previous study and thought there might be enough information in that data set to explore that topic. The majority of the women in this group were recruited from a breast cancer support group so we anticipated that at some point, they had experience with a community support group, a hospital-based support, or both. Our initial steps were to download the interviews of the women with breast cancer and construct a table to capture women's responses to whether a hospital-based support group or community support group was used at any time during or after treatment for breast cancer. We also wanted to capture these women's responses to their experiences with these support groups. Working collaboratively, Melissa and I analyzed the data and presented the findings in the four related themes. These themes described the experiences of these African American breast cancer survivors' experiences with hospital-based support groups and reasons why community support groups were more desirable. Melissa disseminated the findings from this qualitative analysis into three poster presentations, one of which received an award. She is now in the process of submitting the findings from her DNP project as a manuscript in a peer-reviewed journal.

As a nurse scientist, I learned a lot from this experience. One lesson learned was that the findings from my research using qualitative methods can be used not only to explain associations among variables but to better understand patient responses to programs implemented in clinical settings. A better understanding of the relevance of implemented programs for diverse populations contributes to the healthcare system's ability to provide optimal care and health outcomes for all patients. A second lesson learned was that DNP students can be educated on SDOH content through the lens of patient experiences in ways not available through other means. Researchers and Clinicians generally focus on social conditions as SDOH conditions, ignoring cultural and social environmental conditions. Explorations of patient experiences enable us to broaden our perspective on those conditions that shape the care given and ultimately health outcomes for diverse patient populations.

Reflection: Student

During this DNP project, I worked with a faculty mentor and subject matter expert who guided my learning and project milestones. A close working relationship with the subject matter expert guided me through the project, data interpretation, and manuscript writing. Although the subject matter expert had previously collected the interviews through clinical/community partners, I had the opportunity to learn from this expert how critical these individuals were to accessing underserved populations, understand the unique perspectives of SDOH affecting health outcomes, and appreciate the impact this work has within the community.

Simulation for Entry- or Advanced-Level Nursing Education

Compassionate Care and Respectful Communication: SDOH and DEI

Wendy Gibbons, Lalita Kaligotla, Beth Ann Swan, Sofia Biller, Isabella Upchurch, and Dejuan Charles

Background

This simulation scenario was prepared in collaboration with students and based on students' reflections about a real experience they encountered during a community, clinical immersion experience. Upon completion of the immersion, students were asked to submit a written assignment reflecting on an experience that they encountered during their immersion and lessons learned from the experience. For this reflective writing assignment, students were provided specific instructions and guidelines to reflect on a "small moment" that they encountered and what larger lessons they drew from it. Students chose to center their reflections on the experience of a patient. This simulation is based on the students' account of what they witnessed and their processing of how the healthcare system could have served the needs of this patient better. Learners will experience structural competency "the ability of healthcare providers and [students] to appreciate how symptoms, clinical problems, diseases and attitudes toward patients, populations, and health systems are influenced by 'upstream' social determinants of health".

Simulation Description

Course name	SDOH/DEI Simulation Scenario: Respectful Communication and Compassionate Care
Location	Emory Nursing Learning Center
Scenario title	SDOH/DEI: Addressing implicit bias, microaggressions, and structural racism in maternity care
Total session/event run time	
Pre-briefing run time	15 min (with trigger warning)

Scenario run time	10 min (and consider 10 min slow motion)	
Debriefing run time	30 min	
Number of participants	4–6	
Learner type	☐ Novice	☐ Advance Beginner ☐ Competent
	☐ Proficient	☐ Expert
Learner level	☐ Nursing Undergraduate	☐ Nursing Graduate (adapt/update)
	☐ Other: potential for practicing nurses	
Patient information		
Name: Brianna Healey	Age: 18	Gender: female
Height: 5′7″	Weight: 175	DOB: 01/02/2004
Provider: South OB/Gyn	Room #: 4	Code Status: Full

Allergies: None

Past Medical History: non-contributory/negative

Past Surgical History: tonsillectomy at age 7

OB History: G1 P0000 at 38 weeks estimated gestational age. Her prenatal care was significant for a positive test for chlamydia at new OB visit with a negative test of cure 8 weeks later. All other labs are normal, negative GBS. She had 2 ultrasounds that confirmed dates and revealed a normal anatomy.

Social History: Brianna Healey is an 18 years ago. African American female who has completed the 11th grade. Her partner/FOB plans to help with the baby, patient's mother is the primary support person and Brianna, and the baby will live with her mother. Brianna has Medicaid insurance and is not currently working.

Medications: Prenatal vitamins

Learner Shift Report: Today is Friday, Ms. Healy (Brianna) was admitted to the hospital Wednesday evening for a medical induction of labor. Brianna is being induced for elevated blood pressure (gestational hypertension). Her last cervical examination was 2–3 cm, 70% effacement, and −3 station. As you enter the room, you notice she is crying, sweating, and stating she is feeling unremitting pain from the contractions. She states she has asked repeatedly for medication to help with the pain from the contractions. Brianna states she was told by the previous nurse that most women do not complain of this much pain when they are only 2–3 cm dilated. She asks you to please help. Her obstetrician stops by and advises her that if she does not make significant cervical change, she will need to have a cesarean delivery. Brianna tells him she is in so much pain and does not know how much longer she can tolerate the contractions without some help. Brianna agrees to an epidural, and you and your nurse preceptor notify the anesthesiologist and prepare the patient and room for the epidural placement.

Evaluation of experience	☐ Paper	☐ Online
Materials used during session	☐ Yes	☐ No
Laminated copy of the shift report		
SP for the laboring patient		
SP for the nurse/student nurse		
Nursing faculty/CRNA student as the anesthesiologist		
IV fluid		
IV tubing		
IV pole		
Simulated IV site on SP patient's arm		

Epidural tray
LDR bed
Fetal monitor
BP cuff
Stool/chair for patient's feet during the procedure

Post-session/Event Requirement/Assignment

Written guided reflection about personal experience/encounter with discrimination:

Ask each student to share a short example of a time that they felt they were discriminated against or treated unfairly. And then ask the following questions:

- How did it feel?
- What sort of an impact did it have on you?
- How did you cope with that experience?
- What did you learn from it?
- Did it change how you treat others? How?

Overall Goal of Session/Event

Learners begin to understand the individual perspectives and healthcare experiences of persons of color and address implicit bias, microaggressions, and structural racism impair communication and compassionate care.

Specific Learning Objectives

At the end of the simulation, participants will be:

- Describe relevant SDOH influences (identify related SDOH pillars) on physical or mental health from scenarios.
- Identify specific behaviors within the scenario that impede inclusive healthcare.
- Identify resources and strategies within your practice facility that specifically address inappropriate and unacceptable behavior (code of conduct).
- Training on how to advocate for the patient and explain how culturally competent and respectful healthcare can influence patient outcomes.
- Identify patient education strategies to help the patient feel empowered to be a self-advocate (is asking for another provider possible, situational awareness).
- Discuss options for students to address SDOH/DEI concerns in real time during and following experience.
- Explore contextual considerations, for example, consequences of speaking up versus not speaking up), differing contexts of rural and urban healthcare, and evidence-based approaches (even if the situation/experience may lead to an initial sense of powerlessness, we can try to advocate for change over time, with greater awareness and persistence).

Brief Summary of Simulation Scenario

The nurse and student have notified the anesthesiologist of Ms. Healey's status and her desire for an epidural. The anesthesiologist is also told Ms. Healey may need a cesarean delivery. The anesthesiologist walks into the room and immediately says he probably can't do the epidural because she's moving too much. The anesthesiologist treats her roughly and does not inform her what he is doing so she is unprepared when he touches her or sticks her with a needle. The anesthesiologist speaks sharply to the patient throughout the procedure criticizing her for movement and not assisting them.

SDOH Pillars Relevant to the Case Include: Social, Cultural, Policy

Knowledge and Skills Needed: Training on microaggressions, health equity, and compassionate care.

Preparation Work Required Before Simulation: Students must complete SDOH Canvas Training Site.

The Deadliest US State to Have a Baby—https://video.vice.com/en_us/video/the-deadliest-us-state-to-have-a-baby/5f441ac21f3552013a5c7385 [33].

Hoffman, K., Trawalter, S., Axt, J., & Oliver, N. (2016). Racial bias in pain assessment and treatment recommendations, and false beliefs about biological differences between blacks and whites. *PNAS, 113*(6). https://www.pnas.org/content/pnas/113/16/4296.full.pdf [25].

Resource Book: Hossain, A. (2021). *The pain gap*. New York: Simon and Schuster [34].

Scenario Setting: A LDR room in a rural county hospital that serves a diverse population.

Pre-Briefing: This is an "observation only" simulation, however, pre-briefing needs to include a warning of potentially triggering behaviors.

- Confidentiality
  - Do not discuss the content of the scenarios following the simulation session to preserve the realism of the scenarios used and to provide an equitable learning experience for each student.
  - Maintain confidentiality with respect to actions, performance of participants, facilitators, and observers.
- Establish a "fiction contract" with participants. The simulation has been made to be as "real" as possible within resource and technology constraints. Participants should try to suspend disbelief and participate fully with an open mind and positive attitude.
- Provide patient information to participants.

Learner Information: As described in the learner shift report.
Patient Information: As described above in the patient information.

Relevant Physical Assessment Information

Neuro: Normal, alert, oriented × 4
Respiratory: resp rate 22, lungs CTA A&P
Cardiovascular: HR 90, RRR w/o murmur
Gastrointestinal: Normal, normal bowel sounds
OB: gravid abdomen, continuous EFM. FHT's 140, moderate variability, + accels, neg decels. Contractions q2–3 min × 60 s, palpate 2–3+. Vertex by Leopold's
Cervical exam 2–3/60%/−3
Urinary: Voiding without assistance or difficulty
Skin: Intact
IV: Patient, L forearm, site clear. Oxytocin for induction infusing at 12 mu/min via a pump
Latest Vital Signs: Temperature: 37.6-90-22 Blood Pressure 142/92

Scenario Progression

State (i.e., initial and time)	Patient parameters (i.e., vital signs and pain level)	Student expectations	Cues/prompts/to help progress scenario
Initial/0–5 min	BP: HR: RR: O2Sat: Temp:		Operator: Faculty:
	BP: HR: RR: O2Sat: Temp:		Operator: Faculty:
	BP: HR: RR: O2Sat: Temp		Operator: Faculty:

Labs/diagnostics/radiology/EKG results available during simulation: N/A.

Equipment/Supplies/Setup/Moulage

Laminated copy of the shift report
SP for the laboring patient
SP for the nurse/student nurse
Nursing faculty/CRNA student as the anesthesiologist
IV fluid

IV tubing
IV pole
Simulated IV site on SP patient's arm
Epidural tray
LDR bed
Fetal monitor
BP cuff
Stool/chair for patient's feet during the procedure

Roles   Scripts for each role and who will play the role

- L&D nurse
- Nursing student
- Patient (SP)
- Anesthesiologist

Debriefing

- Reinforce that information is confidential and for the purpose of learning.
- How did it feel?
  - Encourage students to express their thoughts or reactions to the scenario.
  - After students express their feelings, guide them to reflective learning.
  - Encourage students to describe SDOH pillars that were uncomfortable for them.
- What went well?
  - If needed and/or time allows, start from the beginning, and talk the group through the experience.
  - Encourage students to reflect on their performance as an individual and, if relevant, as a team/leader/follower.
  - Reinforce positive behaviors.
  - Use concrete examples and outcomes as the basis for inquiry and discussion.
  - Encourage students to ask questions or clarifications of application of SDOH pillars in their assessment and proposed interventions.
- Review objectives and ask students how they met the objectives.
- What could be done differently?
  - If they were to encounter this situation in clinical practice, what would they do differently?
- "Take-aways"
  - Lessons learned from the simulation experience
  - "A-HA" moments
- Close debriefing
  - Acknowledge everyone's participation
  - Thank participants

Other Debriefing Guided Questions

- How did you feel throughout the simulation experience?
- Describe the objectives you were able to achieve.
- Which objectives were you unable to achieve (if any)?
- Did you have the knowledge and skills to meet objectives?
- Were you satisfied with your ability to work through the simulation?
- To Observer: Could the nurses have handled any aspects of the simulation differently?
- What did the team feel was the primary nursing diagnosis?
- How were physical and mental health aspects interrelated in this case?
- *How were SDOH pillars interrelated?*
- Identify takeaways/insights on differential experiences of patients in navigating the healthcare system (depending on socioeconomic and demographic characteristics, or depending on health/disease conditions, etc.)
- Discuss ways in which healthcare professionals can work to create more inclusive and equitable conditions in healthcare systems.
- What were the key assessments and interventions?
- Is there anything else you would like to discuss?

AACN Essentials

Domains/Competencies/Sub-competencies
Domain 2: Person-Centered Care

2.1 Engage with the individual in establishing a caring relationship.
    2.1a Demonstrate qualities of empathy.
    2.1b Demonstrate compassionate care.
    2.1c Establish mutual respect with the individual and family.
2.2 Communicate effectively with individuals.
    2.2a Demonstrate relationship-centered care.
    2.2b Consider individual beliefs, values, and personalized information in communications.
    2.2c Use a variety of communication modes appropriate for the context.
    2.2d Demonstrate the ability to conduct sensitive or difficult conversations.
    2.2f Demonstrate emotional intelligence in communications.

Domain 5: Quality and Safety

5.3 Contribute to a culture of provider and work environment safety.
    5.3d Recognize one's role in sustaining a just culture reflecting civility and respect.

Domain 6: Interprofessional Partnerships

6.1 Communicate in a manner that facilitates a partnership approach to quality care delivery.

      6.1d Articulate impact of diversity, equity, and inclusion on team-based communications.

      6.1e Communicate individual information in a professional, accurate, and timely manner.

6.4 Work with other professions to maintain a climate of mutual learning, respect, and shared values.

      6.4c Engage in constructive communication to facilitate conflict management.

Domain 9: Professionalism

9.2 Employ a participatory approach to nursing care.

      9.2b Facilitate health and healing through compassionate caring.

      9.2d Advocate for practices that advance diversity, equity, and inclusion.

      9.2e Demonstrate cultural sensitivity and humility in practice.

9.6 Integrate diversity, equity, and inclusion as core to one's professional identity.

      9.6a Demonstrate respect for diverse individual differences and diverse communities and populations.

      9.6b Demonstrate awareness of personal and professional values and conscious and unconscious biases.

      9.6c Integrate core principles of social justice and human rights into practice.

Concepts

Communication
Compassionate Care
Diversity, Equity, and Inclusion
Social Determinants of Health

Reflection: Student, Sofia Biller

"I can't do this anymore."

A drop of sweat rolled down from a black curl on the laboring woman's forehead as she gripped the bedside rails hard enough for the blood to turn her fingers dark red.

Thirty minutes after calling, the anesthesiologist finally entered the room in an exasperated huff, as if we called him away from his job. He rolled his eyes after glancing at the trembling patient. From the moment he walked into the room, I was fairly certain the epidural wouldn't be successful. Not because he's not good at his job, but because he didn't want it to work. The patient's pain, shaking, and shallow breathing were a clear inconvenience for him.

"I can't do this if you're not sitting still!" he yelled at the young Black woman, the nurses becoming quiet and wide eyed. Any bit of equanimity the patient had now dissipated.

The uncomfortable energy in the room seemed to encourage the anesthesiologist to do his job. He approached the young Black woman, whose whole body was now vibrating in pain, from behind as one of the nurses helped her into a position for the procedure.

Trying to calm the young Black woman, I held her by the shoulders, encouraging her to mirror my breaths. Soon her forehead was against mine and her body slowly became still. I could feel the sweat from her brow, cautious of my own position and hoping I wouldn't move and disturb her calm. We breathed in unison.

As the anesthesiologist began preparing the sterile procedure, he rolled his eyes at every small movement the patient made and glared at the nurses in hopes for one of us to call the procedure off ourselves. But we're nurses after all, and no sound nurse would let their patient exist in the amount of pain this woman was experiencing. So, despite the dirty looks and hesitancy, the anesthesiologist began his procedure, draping a sheer plastic sheet over her back, attaching long needles to syringes, giving the patient little information as to what he was doing. She was powerless.

"You're going to feel a pinch now. Don't move."

My heart now beating out of my chest, I did all I could to keep her in position. I knew we were out of warnings, and the anesthesiologist would stop the procedure at her next jolt.

"My leg!" She exclaimed when he began weaving the catheter down her spine.

"Don't move." The doctor snapped.

"You're so strong." I whispered quietly.

She exhaled and the catheter continued. Her shoulders weakened against my hands.

As the anesthesiologist began taping the tubing to the patient's body, I could tell he was not confident in the epidural's success.

"You may have been moving too much for this to work." He said, still behind the patient.

The woman let out an exasperated breath. Blamed for the procedure's failure and hopelessness, she could not form words to describe her pain and emotions. With a final eye roll, the anesthesiologist left, the girl still shaking in my arms. The room fell silent.

What did I just witness?

The patient opted for a c-section after 20 min of no relief or alternative pain management recommendations. The epidural didn't work.

The anesthesiologist went about his day, confident, I'm sure, in his technique and care. The following epidural he placed was across the hall. A dirty blonde, mid-20-year old sat with her eyes closed, breathing slowly waiting for relief from her frequent contractions. The anesthesiologist placed a hand on her shaking leg as he explained the procedure. I could still hear wailing from across the way as nurses prepped the patient for her c-section. In about 20 min, the anesthesiologist was finished with the freckled woman, taking her vital signs, and asking how she was feeling. The epidural worked.

I'm not sure if the epidural would've ever worked with the young Black woman, but I do know that she was never given a chance. Systemic racism, implicit bias, and microaggressions were displayed within seconds of the provider entering the room, and when faced with this at the moment, myself and the nurses became paralyzed, unsure of our position with respect to the anesthesiologist.

He got what he wanted. The patient wouldn't listen, she couldn't understand what it was that he was doing, so why explain it? She couldn't keep it together long enough for the procedure. Yes, she was having contractions, but what does that matter? He does this procedure multiple times a day, it can't be his problem to make her comfortable. And with that he got what he wanted, the epidural did not work. The patient could not be treated.

Reflection: Student, Dejuan Charles

I found myself on autopilot walking through the long monotone hallways of Colquitt County Regional Hospital, my first time in a rural hospital other than where I grew up. It was familiar yet different simply because most of the patients were not Black. The one Black patient I saw was an 18-year-old woman who was in labor for 3 days with failure to progress. I felt like I had to give special attention to the amount of pain she was in.

I greeted her and introduced myself only to be met with a moan of pain and incoherent sentences. Fair enough I said to myself, I went to get her some ice chips and water while she awaited an epidural. In comes the anesthesiologist, a white male with a worn-out disposition. It felt off the way he lazily strolled into the room, barely attempting to converse with this woman and explain his process in a calm manner. Instead, she was met with quick imperative instructions. Upon noticing how much pain she was in, I thought that I would get to see how a doctor works around such an obstacle, but I only witnessed impatience and a lack of sympathy that you would expect in a child. To a woman clearly convulsing from pain he loudly proclaimed, "If you keep moving like this there is no way I will be able to get this in, you need to stay still!" he shouted at roughly 7 am. She attempted to remain still while experiencing this pain but as soon as he touched her lower back, unannounced I might add, she instinctively flinched. He rolled his eyes, dropped his marking pen, and yelled at her "YOU ARE DONE, WE ARE DONE, I CANNOT DO THIS IF YOU KEEP MOVING LIKE THIS," followed by a sigh of frustration. Sofia and I quickly exchanged looks of confusion as what we were witnessing was drastically different from any patient interactions we had witnessed. I thought that this was one of the moments that drastically changes a patient's outcome. It is not the type of care that this man delivers to all his patients, I was sure of it. It felt as though he was judging her for all kinds of things like her age, her skin color, and maybe even the circumstances that brought her here. As she tried to hold still, embracing the nurse confronting her to relieve some pain, the procedure was complete but was ineffective. Did he do it wrong? Did he rush this procedure? Did he know that he rushed this procedure and/or failed it? These were all the questions that rattled my brain as I saw how she made the crushing decision to have major surgery to get the baby out at 18 years old. I felt responsible at that moment because I knew there was something I could have done. I could have been a better patient advocate, tried getting her heat packs, I could have tried getting her to walk, aromatherapy, repositioning, anything that could have helped ease the pain and maybe could have helped her progress. I didn't get to see the birth, which was another heartbreak in itself as that woman's mother was asking Sofia where I'd disappeared to. I knew she was looking for another face similar to hers, a black face to give her comfort in a clearly uncomfortable situation. We know that people of color often are mistreated in the medical setting and although I failed to assuage her from this reality, I now know how to identify situations like this and intervene appropriately so that all patients receive adequate healthcare.

Reflection: Student, Isabella Upchurch

Colquitt County Regional Hospital is a regional perinatal center located in a very rural area of Georgia. Given this hospital's regional location, there are fewer options for perinatal care for patients residing further away from the center. This means that it could potentially take some patients hours of travel to access perinatal care. In addition, the inability to take time off from work, and similar factors prevent a large number of people from accessing needed healthcare. The Ellenton Clinic is a federally funded rural primary healthcare clinic based in Colquitt County, where many migrant farmworkers who work on the farms spread out across this county, go to access perinatal and primary care. In the absence of this federally funded clinic, many patients in this region would receive no perinatal or primary care. If more clinics like the Ellenton Clinic existed in rural communities in Georgia, then it could lead to significantly better perinatal outcomes due to increased access to healthcare.

References

1. American Association of Colleges of Nursing. The essentials: core competencies for professional nursing education. American Association of Colleges of Nursing; 2021.
2. Coyne I. Families and health-care professionals' perspectives and expectations of family-centered care: hidden expectations and unclear roles. Health Expect. 2015;18(5):796–808. https://doi.org/10.1111/hex.12104.
3. World Health Organization. Social determinants of health; n.d.. https://www.who.int/health-topics/social-determinants-of-health#tab=tab_1. Accessed 20 May 2022.
4. Institute for Patient- and Family-Centered Care [IPFCC]. Patient- and family-centered care; n.d. https://www.ipfcc.org/about/pfcc.html. Accessed 24 May 2022.
5. Robert Wood Johnson Foundation. Catalysts for change: harnessing the power of nurses to build population health in the 21st century. Executive summary. Princeton, NJ; 2017.
6. National League for Nursing. NLN releases a vision for integration of the social determinants of health into nursing education curricula. Nurs Educ Perspect. 2019;40(6):390. https://doi.org/10.1097/01.NEP.0000000000000597.
7. Robertson B, Brasher S, Wright P. An approach to integrating social determinants of health in an accelerated prelicensure academic-practice partnership program. Nurs Educ. 2021;47(2):130. https://doi.org/10.1097/NNE.0000000000001111.
8. Thornton M, Persaud S. Preparing today's nurses: social determinants of health and nursing education. Online J Issues Nurs. 2018;23(3)
9. Muirhead L, Brasher S, Broadnax D, Chandler R. A framework for evaluating SDOH curriculum integration. J Prof Nurs. 2022;39:1–9. https://doi.org/10.1016/j.profnurs.2021.12.004.
10. Riquino MR, Nguyen VL, Reese SE, Molloy J. Using a transdiagnostic perspective to disrupt White supremacist applications of the DSM. Adv Soc Work. 2021;21(2/3):750–65. https://doi.org/10.18060/24049.
11. Fadus MC, Ginsburg KR, Sobowale K, Halliday-Boykins CA, Bryant BE, Gray KM, Squeglia LM. Unconscious bias and the diagnosis of disruptive behavior disorders and ADHD in African

American and Hispanic youth. Acad Psychiatr. 2020;44(1):95–102. https://doi.org/10.1007/s40596-019-01127-6.

12. Inker LA, Eneanya ND, Coresh J, Tighiouart H, Wang D, Sang Y, et al. New creatinine-and cystatin C–based equations to estimate GFR without race. N Engl J Med. 2021;385(19):1737–49.

13. Miller WG, Kaufman HW, Levey AS, Straseski JA, Wilhelms KW, Yu HY, et al. National Kidney Foundation Laboratory Engagement Working Group recommendations for implementing the CKD-EPI 2021 race-free equations for estimated glomerular filtration rate: practical guidance for clinical laboratories. Clin Chem. 2022;68(4):511–20.

14. Ifekwunigwe JO, Wagner JK, Yu JH, Harrell TM, Bamshad MJ, Royal CD. A qualitative analysis of how anthropologists interpret the race construct. Am Anthropol. 2017;119(3):422–34. https://doi.org/10.1111/aman.12890.

15. Alvarez-Arango S, Ogunwole SM, Sequist TD, Burk CM, Blumenthal KG. Vancomycin infusion reaction—moving beyond "red man syndrome". N Engl J Med. 2021;384(14):1283–6.

16. National Institutes of Health. National Institutes of Health revitalization act of 1993: clinical research equity regarding women and minorities. 1993.

17. Zucker I, Prendergast BJ. Sex differences in pharmacokinetics predict adverse drug reactions in women. Biol Sex Differ. 2020;11:1–14. https://doi.org/10.1186/s13293-020-00308-5.

18. Perry B. What happened to you? Conversations on trauma, resilience, and healing. Flatiron Books: An Oprah Book; 2021.

19. Castillo MH, Pabon TA. Children of the land. New York: Harper; 2020.

20. Angelou M. I know why the cage bird sings. London: Virago; 2015.

21. Patterson J, Eversman M, Mooney C. Walk in my combat boots: true stories from America's bravest warriors. Little, Brown, and Company; 2021.

22. American Nurses Association. Code of ethics for nurses with interpretive statements. 2015. https://www.nursingworld.org/coe-view-only

23. Hamilton JB. Integrating social determinants of health into the emory nursing curriculum [powerpoint slides]. Emory University Nell Hodgson Woodruff School of Nursing; 2019.

24. Baird C. EthicsGame™: ethics education transformed. 2022. https://www.ethicsgame.com/exec/site/about_us.html

25. Hoffman KM, Trawalter S, Axt JR, Oliver MN. Racial bias in pain assessment and treatment recommendations, and false beliefs about biological differences between blacks and whites. Proc Natl Acad Sci USA. 2016;113(16):4296–301.

26. Compton P, Blacher S. Nursing education in the midst of the opioid crisis. Pain Manag Nursing. 2020;21(1):35–42.

27. Pasero C, Quinlan-Colwell A, Rae D, Broglio K, Drew D. American Society for Pain Management Nursing position statement: prescribing and administering opioid doses based solely on pain intensity. Pain Manag Nurs. 2016;17(3):170–80.

28. Wideman TH, Edwards RR, Walton DM, Martel MO, Hudon A, Seminowicz DA. The multimodal assessment model of pain: a novel framework for further integrating the subjective pain experience within research and practice. Clin J Pain. 2019;35(3):212.

29. Healthy People 2030. https://health.gov/healthypeople.

30. National Institute on Minority Health and Health Disparities (NIMHD). NIMHD research framework. 2017. https://nimhd.nih.gov/researchFramework. Accessed 9 May 2022.

31. National Institute of Nursing Research. National Institute of Nursing Research 2022–2026 strategic plan. 2022. https://www.ninr.nih.gov/sites/files/docs/NINR_One-Pager12_508c.pdf. Accessed 9 May 2022.

32. Kris MG, Johnson BE, Berry LD, Kwiatkowski DJ, Iafrate AJ, Wistuba II, Varella-Garcia M, Franklin WA, Aronson SL, Su PF, Shyr Y, Camidge DR, Sequist LV, Glisson BS, Khuri FR, Garon EB, Pao W, Rudin C, Schiller J, Haura EB, et al. Using multiplexed assays of oncogenic drivers in lung cancers to select targeted drugs. JAMA. 2014;311(19):1998–2006. https://doi.org/10.1001/jama.2014.3741.

33. The Deadliest U.S. State to have a baby. https://video.vice.com/en_us/video/the-deadliest-us-state-to-have-a-baby/5f441ac21f3552013a5c7385

34. Hossain A. The pain gap. New York: Simon and Schuster; 2021.

Evaluating Social Determinants of Health Integration in Nursing Curricula

6

Lisa Muirhead, Susan Brasher, Rasheeta Chandler, and Laura P. Kimble

Learning Objectives

1. Objective 1: Describe approaches to evaluation of SDOH integration into educational programs within the nursing and health professions.
2. Objective 2: Discuss the relevance of nurses' social accountability in responding to societal needs.
3. Objective 3: Describe an exemplar of a structured SDOH curriculum evaluation model.
4. Objective 4: Identify SDOH evaluation model(s) that is/are applicable to varied educational institutions.

Introduction

Curricular innovation is an imperative within the discipline of nursing as the challenges in providing nursing care to patients are created by societal changes as well as changes within the nursing profession. It is critical that nursing students be prepared to deliver high quality, cost-effective care within a contemporary healthcare environment, where, unfortunately, health inequities exist and persist. Nursing faculty are integral to helping students understand the social determinants of health (SDOH) and the structures that perpetuate health inequities [1] and preparing students to care for those experiencing health disparities at the individual, community, and population levels [2, 3]. In this chapter, we provide a brief overview around SDOH integration into nursing and health professions described within the literature with a focus on evaluation approaches. Building on the foundational concept of

L. Muirhead (✉) · S. Brasher · R. Chandler · L. P. Kimble
Nell Hodgson Woodruff School of Nursing, Emory University, Atlanta, GA, USA
e-mail: Lisa.muirhead@emory.edu; Susan.brasher@emory.edu;
Rasheeta.chander@emory.edu; lkimble@emory.edu

© The Author(s), under exclusive license to Springer Nature Switzerland AG 2023
J. B. Hamilton et al. (eds.), *Integrating a Social Determinants of Health Framework into Nursing Education*, https://doi.org/10.1007/978-3-031-21347-2_6

social accountability in nursing, we provide an evaluative approach to SDOH curriculum integration inclusive of an assessment obtained from both faculty and students. The chapter concludes with a presentation of the framework we used to guide our evaluation process and inform refinement of our approach as well as suggestions for other models of evaluation that nursing institutions might consider using within their programs.

Multiple instances were reported of integrating SDOH concepts into nursing curricula [4–8] and health care professions such as medicine [9–11], and dentistry [12]. Within medicine, SDOH integration appeared to be embedded within specialties such as pediatrics [11], psychiatry [11], and emergency medicine [13], or specific foci such as health advocacy [9, 14]. A scoping review of undergraduate medical education SDOH integration [15] revealed multiple different approaches to SDOH curriculum integration to support student learning and competencies, however, the literature lacked specificity which made synthesizing the evidence highly challenging. For nursing specifically, the scope of SDOH integration ranged from comprehensive SDOH integration within an entire college [5] to use of gaming within an elective course on primary care [7]. Davis and colleagues [5] primarily focused on diversity, equity, and inclusion as SDOH was integrated within the nursing curriculum across pre-licensure and graduate curricula. They were distinctive because they also described SDOH at the PhD in Nursing curricular level. With a focus on experiential learning, they used existing frameworks to guide integration such as the Simulation in PhD Programs (SIPP©) framework. They acknowledged their next steps would be developing a framework to guide standardization of evaluation measures.

Porter and colleagues [6] described how they integrated SDOH within a concept-based pre-licensure curriculum. Examples of multiple individual and group learning activities were provided across a wide array of individual nursing courses, however, they did not discuss evaluation of the integration among individual students or the courses in which the SDOH learning activities were offered. Within graduate nursing education, Buys & Somerall [4], described an innovative longitudinal three phase assignment within a family nurse practitioner clinical course, where students conducted a SDOH literature review, prepared a screening tool for SDOH relevant to their clinical setting, and then conducted 100 SDOH screenings or 50 referrals by the end of the semester. They implemented evaluation measures that included student course evaluations that measured perceived knowledge of SDOH, importance of SDOH screening, and intention to integrate SDOH screenings and referrals into their future clinical practice. They reported that students' perceptions of the SDOH-related learning activity changed from initial perceptions that the activity was "busy work" to belief that the assignment truly helped them understand the determinants of health. Along with the student evaluation data, Buys and Somerall [4] stated their desire to examine longer-term student learning outcomes beyond the bounds of that single clinical course.

Schroeder and colleagues [8] focused on service learning and community engagement as experiential learning for students to learn about the SDOH. Using a flipped classroom approach, they provided didactic content along with active learning strategies for students to gain foundational knowledge in SDOH before completing clinical activities within the community focused on health promotion with a final course outcome of a health promotion project. Evaluation approaches within the course included collecting survey data from students about their knowledge of SDOH and how they intended to apply SDOH in clinical experiences.

Overall, the literature within nursing and the health professions emphasized the need for robust evaluation methods that truly measure the impact of SDOH curricular integration [15]. It is important to consider how SDOH is profoundly related to what Sharma and colleagues [16] call the social determinants of health equity (SDOE). They emphasize the goal of education around SDOH should be to bring about a fundamental change in the way students think and engage in clinical practice so that they are committed to advancing health equity [16]. This perspective is closely related to the concept of social accountability and how nursing education should be held accountable for meeting social needs.

Social Accountability in Nursing Education

As the national emphasis on addressing the social determinants of health continues to expand, it is important that schools of nursing recognize their social accountability in meeting population needs, including social needs, in nursing education. One of the World Health Organization's [17] seminal papers calling for accountability in medical education, elaborates on the values and importance of social accountability in responding to societal needs and uses these conceptual lenses in evaluating sustained progress toward accountability goals [17]. Social accountability is considered the institutional obligation to address the needs of those they intend to serve in society [17–19]. The obligation requires intentional aims in domains of education, research, and service that advance efforts in meeting the prioritized health needs of populations [17]. A social accountability framework has direct implications for nursing education in developing and evaluating curricula that acknowledge nurses' role in addressing social determinants of health and prepare nursing graduates with a deep understanding of their accountability to the public's health and the transformative power they possess to intervene and impact health outcomes within health systems. While social responsibility implies awareness of duty to respond and is often referenced in schools of nursing, social accountability focuses on measurable outcomes and supports evaluative efforts on progress toward meeting societal needs [19–21].

The World Health Organization identifies four values that educational institutions can use to measure progress toward social accountability including relevance, quality, cost-effectiveness, and equity in health care. Relevance is the extent to which content and context are given high priority in education, research, and service [17]. In education, this may include structured curricula with didactic and experiential learning pedagogy in community-based settings that make the connection between social issues and health, as well as the importance of social accountability and advocacy. Importance is given to addressing high-priority needs and gaps in services within communities. A broad spectrum of longitudinal educational offerings is purposively focused on stages of learning experiences that build upon knowledge with an advancing level of application in practice [19, 21]. Opportunities for reflective activities, perspective taking, and value clarification can be used to expand students' capacity for community engagement. Developing curriculum objectives with the participation of community partners and inviting patient partners into classrooms to share their life experiences represents a conscious effort to be socially accountable. Patient partners in clinical settings can also serve as evaluators of students' skills in addressing social determinants of health [21]. The values of social accountability can be represented in formulating task forces for curriculum design and evaluation that addresses high-priority health needs of populations along with strong professional development of faculty and staff [17, 19]. While quality may be contextually different in various countries, the social accountability value of high-quality care is evidence-based, comprehensive, and take into consideration what is acceptable and expected by consumers of care, culturally and socially [17, 19]. Cost-effective describes the best use of resources to deliver high-quality care, and the collaborative research efforts between government, private sector stakeholders, and schools to examine the use of resources and their effectiveness on care delivery [17, 19].

As a fundamental tenet to social accountability, equity ensures that all people have access to high-quality health care through all levels of health systems [17, 19]. These values are equally important within the domains of education, research, and service as depicted in Fig. 6.1 and provides an implicit foundation for interventions that evaluate nursing educational efforts that make relevant the interrelationship among social and structural forces and health. To be socially accountable infers that addressing the social determinants of health to achieve health equity is not a choice within nursing, but nursing's obligation to society.

Fig. 6.1 Social accountability and domains of institutional responsibility

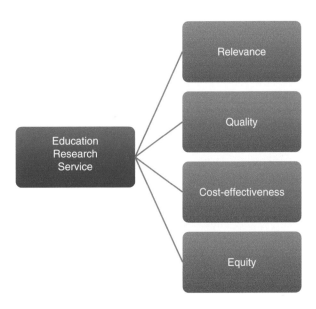

Overview of SDOH Integration

Systemic integration and evaluation of SDOH were piloted first in the pre-licensure nursing program prior to expanding to the post-licensure programs. Beginning in curriculum committee, pre-licensure faculty, and program directors were asked to assess SDOH integration in the current curriculum based on the following criteria: didactic content, trending topics relative to SDOH, pedagogical strategies, and experiential learning activities through simulation and clinical activities [22]. A team of faculty experts consisting of Diversity, Equity, and Inclusion (DEI) leadership, and tenure and clinical track faculty, convened as the SDOH evaluation team to develop an evaluation plan that would assess faculty and student knowledge, skills, confidence, and perceived relevance of SDOH.

Faculty Evaluation

Faculty surveys were developed by the SDOH evaluation team and beta tested by the curriculum committee to elicit feedback on readability and content suggestions (i.e., items that were omitted). Final surveys were then distributed to all faculty to assess their perceived preparation and confidence in teaching SDOH, as well as the extent to which they were integrating SDOH into their course, additional training needs, and their perceived relevance of SDOH to their clinical practice, service role, and research. Additional demographic information was included in the survey, such as:

- Age range (e.g., 25–30 and 31–35)
- Racial and ethnic background
- Track and rank (e.g., Clinical track, Tenure Track, and Assistant Professor)
- Program of study primarily teach (e.g., Pre-licensure BSN and Post-licensure DNP)

Student Evaluation

Student surveys were developed by the SDOH evaluation team and deployed to pre-licensure nursing students to assess their perceived relevance of SDOH with respect to the nurse's role in assessing and addressing SDOH. Students were asked to rate 0–4 the relevance of various Social, Cultural, Environmental, and Policy conditions surrounding SDOH. Examples of these conditions include the following:

- *Social Conditions*—Access to education, financial resources, employment opportunities, social support, language and health literacy, access to preventative health services, and incarceration history.
- *Cultural Conditions*—Military background status, religion/spirituality, cultural customs and beliefs, interpersonal racism/microaggressions, gender identity, sexual orientation, and ethnic identity.

- *Environmental Conditions (Physical and Social Environments)*—Access to safe and habitable living space, access to foods that support healthy eating patterns, exposure to toxins, migrant/seasonal/agricultural work, air quality, supportive relationships with family, social capital, access to faith-based institutions, access to health care settings, quality of schools/academic settings, access to recreational facilities, worksites/schools recreational settings, safe and quality housing, safe neighborhood, safety and violence risk, and access to affordable transportation.
- *Policy Conditions*—Insurance status, access to abortion services (reproductive justice), access to family planning, firearm policies, education/housing policies, civil rights, LGBTQIA rights, housing laws, recreational drug use and laws, and child protection laws.

An additional student survey was developed by the SDOH evaluation survey and deployed to pre-licensure nursing students to evaluate their knowledge, skills, and confidence in assessing and addressing SDOH in terms of Social, Cultural, Environmental, and Policy conditions. Knowledge, skills, and confidence were measured separately, as well as assessing and addressing these conditions knowing that some students may feel more confident, knowledgeable, and skilled to assess versus address. Additionally, it was important for the SDOH evaluation team to identify where students have most confidence, knowledge, and skills, to identify potential curricular gaps and learning opportunities.

Course Evaluation

Survey questions to evaluate SDOH course integration were built into anonymous end-of-semester student course evaluations. Students were asked to evaluate the extent to which the course emphasized SDOH across Social Conditions, Cultural Conditions, Environmental Conditions, and Policy. Additionally, students were asked to rate the faculty's expertise in integrating SDOH into the course on a five-point Likert scale.

Exemplar: Social Determinants of Health (SDOH) Curriculum Integration Evaluation Model

Many schools of nursing are anticipating changes in accreditation standards that align with the new competency-based Essentials for nursing education. Curriculums are being reformed to reflect the integration of social determinants of health but to fully actualize substantial and sustained changes in nursing education, it is important to evaluate programmatic efforts. An evaluative process provides necessary knowledge relative to the strength of innovation and encourages accountability [23]. Kirkpatrick's model distinguishes four progressive levels of evaluating training programs within organizations (see Fig. 6.2). The four levels include reaction, learning,

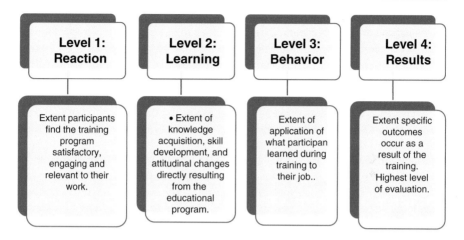

Fig. 6.2 The Kirkpatrick training evaluation model

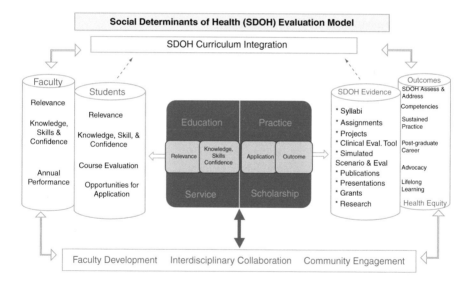

Fig. 6.3 Social Determinants of Health (SDOH) Evaluation Model [22]

behavior, and results. As evaluation progresses from one level to the next, it becomes more complex and meaningful [24].

The Social Determinants of Health (SDOH) Curriculum Integration Evaluation Model (Fig. 6.3) illustrates the four domains that can be impacted by integration of SDOH within nursing curricula inclusive of education, practice, service, and scholarship, and similar to the domains of the WHO's social accountability framework. The model depicts the use of the four levels of Kirkpatrick's model to appraise nursing students' perception of relevance of SDOH to nursing practice; knowledge, skills, and confidence in assessing and addressing SDOH; use of course evaluations to appraise students' perceived satisfaction and extent of course delivery of SDOH concepts; and experiential learning opportunities to test SDOH knowledge and skill acquisition through application. The model mirrors the approach used for student evaluation in appraising faculty perception of relevance of teaching the SDOH in their respective area of expertise; knowledge, skills, and confidence in teaching and contextualizing the SDOH to course content, concepts, and integration in a myriad of pedagogical approaches; and opportunity to discuss the application of SDOH in education, practice, scholarship, and service during an annual performance review. The barrels to the right of the domains for impact illustrate the several types of exemplars of evidence of curriculum integration and implementation outcomes. Thus, reflecting pedagogical approaches to advance knowledge of SDOH constructs and ultimately advance goals toward health equity. The model also reflects the feedback loop of student and faculty evaluation on informing curriculum integration, faculty development, interdisciplinary collaboration, community engagement, and program outcomes.

Alternative Models of Evaluation

Exemplars of models that were integrated into one institution's effort to have a systematic approach to evaluating SDOH curricular integration have been described in earlier sections of this chapter; however, there is value in knowing alternative models that can inform evaluation [25]. Schools of Nursing vary in size, culture, mission, goals, and infrastructure, thus, scrutiny of various models is essential to employ the appropriate evaluation mechanism for the SDOH curricula integration of diverse nursing schools. Table 6.1 provides a list of models that can be considered as alternative options for evaluating SDOH curricula integration.

Table 6.1 Exemplars of evaluation models

Model	Model description	Model constructs and processes
Implementation outcomes [26]	Evaluating the effects of deliberate and purposive actions to implement new treatments, practices, and services	Acceptability, adoption, appropriateness, feasibility, fidelity, implementation cost, penetration, and sustainability
RE-AIM [27]	Reach: Proportion of the population who participated in the intervention Efficacy: Defined as positive outcomes minus negative outcomes Adoption: Proportion of settings, practices, and plans that will adopt this intervention Implementation: Extent to which the intervention is implemented as intended in the real world Maintenance: Extent to which the program is sustained over time	Reach, efficacy, adoption, implementation, and maintenance

Table 6.1 (continued)

Model	Model description	Model constructs and processes
CIPP evaluation Model [28, 29]	An evaluation model was created for the decision-making toward education improvement	Context, input, process, and product
Competency-based evaluation models [30]	Evaluation of a curriculum based on a set of competencies Six steps to more effective program and curriculum evaluation: 1. Evaluating the alignment of the program mission with defined outcomes 2. Program curriculum mapping to a set of competencies 3. Competencies mapped to course objectives 4. Establish competency measures with summative and formative evaluation strategies 5. Synthesizing results of summative assessment to appraise student learning outcomes relative to competencies 6. Create an action plan for program curriculum improvement to strengthen competencies	Alignment, mapping competencies, competency measures, summative and formative evaluation, and program improvement plan
Phillips' model of learning evaluation [31]	Builds on Kirkpatrick's Four-Level Model of Learning Evaluation by adding concepts related to return on investment (ROI) of training to evaluate benefits and cost of training	Reaction, learning, behavior, results, return on investment
Purpose evaluation [32]	An evaluation model that focuses on the purpose of evaluation	Goals-based, process-based, and outcome-based
Typology of program evaluation framework [33]	The framework defines central purposes and stages of evaluation Purposes focus on program assessment and improvement. Stages focus on the process and outcomes of the program. Formative and summative evaluations may be used to appraise achievements, implementation, and contribute to overall program improvement	Assessment, improvement, process, outcome

Conclusion

Integral to embedding SDOH concepts in nursing education curricula is a deliberate plan to evaluate outcomes associated with this effort. While these undertakings require substantive allocation of resources and time, the resulting information drives sustainable change that contributes to program quality. Scaling evaluation plans to appraise SDOH curriculum integration should consider changes over time for individual students as they progress through programs and demonstrate competencies to assess and address SDOH from both didactic and clinical teaching strategies. Notably, integration of experiential learning versus didactic learning requires different pedagogical approaches for incorporating SDOH. Thus, leveraging varied opportunities to deepen understanding relative to how social and structural forces influence health and health outcomes. Additional curriculum integration metrics involve surveying graduates about their professional practice and the extent of addressing SDOH among individual patients, families, and communities, and graduates' involvement in policy development at a micro or macro level within health systems. Moving beyond institutional-focused SDOH evaluation to evaluating nursing practice that is well aligned with national practice standards and educational frameworks is essential to overall efforts to advance health equity.

Chapter Review Questions

The College of Nursing of Ashland University (fictitious name) has integrated the SDOH in the major clinical courses across the pre-licensure, advanced practice, and Doctor of Nursing Practice programs; however, the faculty have not yet begun integration into core courses such as pharmacology and pathophysiology. To date, the focus of the evaluation has been on students' end-of-course ratings of knowledge around the social determinants of health.

Question 1: Which of the following actions are least likely to contribute to robust evaluation within the School of Nursing:

(A) Identifying an evaluation framework to inform approaches.
(B) Conducting a longitudinal evaluation of how students' perceptions of SDOH change over time in their programs of study.
(C) Conducting a faculty forum to gain consensus around what SDOH components should be taught in didactic and clinical courses.
(D) Expanding evaluation indicators to include perceptions of SDOH integration by students from clinical partners.

Correct answer: (C) Gaining consensus around what SDOH components should be taught within didactic and clinical courses is important but should be completed prior to curriculum integration being undertaken.

Question 2: What is the major disadvantage of using knowledge of SDOH at one point in time as the major approach to evaluating SDOH curricular integration:

(A) Knowledge of SDOH is easy to promote among nursing students and not worthwhile to measure.
(B) Knowledge of SDOH does not necessarily mean that nursing students will apply that knowledge.
(C) Measuring knowledge of SDOH is complicated and time consuming.
(D) None of the above.

Answer: (B) It is important that students gain knowledge of the SDOH, however, evaluating how students use or apply the SDOH concepts and how this knowledge improves over time are stronger evaluation approaches.

References

1. Murray TA. Teaching the social and structural determinants of health: considerations for faculty. J Nurs Educ. 2021;60(2):63–4. https://doi.org/10.3928/01484834-20210120-01.
2. Scott PN, Davis A, Gray LE, Jeffs DA, Lefler LL. Imperatives for integrating culture of health concepts into nursing education. J Nurs Educ. 2020;59(11):605–9. https://doi.org/10.3928/01484834-20201020-02.
3. Younas A, Shahzad S. Emphasizing the need to integrate and teach sociocultural determinants of health in undergraduate nursing curricula. Nurse Educ Today. 2021;103:104943. https://doi.org/10.1016/j.nedt.2021.104943.
4. Buys KC, Somerall D. Social determinants of health screening and referral: innovation in graduate nursing education. J Nurs Educ. 2018;57(9):571–2. https://doi.org/10.3928/01484834-20180815-13.
5. Davis VH, Murillo C, Chappell KK, et al. Tipping point: integrating social determinants of health concepts in a college of nursing. J Nurs Educ. 2021;60(12):703–6. https://doi.org/10.3928/01484834-20211004-05.
6. Porter K, Jackson G, Clark R, Waller M, Stanfill AG. Applying social determinants of health to nursing education using a concept-based approach. J Nurs Educ. 2020;59(5):293–6. https://doi.org/10.3928/01484834-20200422-12.
7. Pollio EW, Patton EM, Nichols LS, Bowers DA. Gamification of primary care in a baccalaureate nursing education program. Nurs Educ Perspect. 2021; https://doi.org/10.1097/01.NEP.0000000000000925.
8. Schroeder K, Garcia B, Phillips RS, Lipman TH. Addressing social determinants of health through community engagement: an undergraduate nursing course. J Nurs Educ. 2019;58(7):423–6. https://doi.org/10.3928/01484834-20190614-07.
9. Boroumand S, Stein MJ, Jay M, Shen JW, Hirsh M, Dharamsi S. Addressing the health advocate role in medical education. BMC Med Educ. 2020;20(1):28. https://doi.org/10.1186/s12909-020-1938-7.
10. Kronsberg H, Bettencourt AF, Vidal C, Platt RE. Education on the social determinants of mental health in child and adolescent psychiatry fellowships. Acad Psychiatry. 2022;46(1):50–4. https://doi.org/10.1007/s40596-020-01269-y.
11. Morrison JM, Marsicek SM, Hopkins AM, Dudas RA, Collins KR. Using simulation to increase resident comfort discussing social determinants of health. BMC Med Educ. 2021;21(1):601. https://doi.org/10.1186/s12909-021-03044-5.
12. Leadbetter D, Holden ACL. How are the social determinants of health being taught in dental education? J Dent Educ. 2021;85(4):539–54. https://doi.org/10.1002/jdd.12487.
13. Moffett SE, Shahidi H, Sule H, Lamba S. Social determinants of health curriculum integrated into a core emergency medicine clerkship. MedEdPORTAL. 2019;15:10789. https://doi.org/10.15766/mep_2374-8265.10789.
14. Hubinette M, Dobson S, Scott I, Sherbino J. Health advocacy. Med Teach. 2017;39(2):128–35. https://doi.org/10.1080/0142159X.2017.1245853.
15. Doobay-Persaud A, Adler MD, Bartell TR, et al. Teaching the social determinants of health in undergraduate medical education: a scoping review. J Gen Intern Med. 2019;34(5):720–30. https://doi.org/10.1007/s11606-019-04876-0.
16. Sharma M, Pinto AD, Kumagai AK. Teaching the social determinants of health: a path to equity or a road to nowhere? Acad Med. 2018;93(1):25–30. https://doi.org/10.1097/ACM.0000000000001689.
17. Boelen C, Heck JE, World Health Organization. Division of Development of Human Resources for Health. Defining and measuring the social accountability of medical schools/Charles Boelen and Jeffery E. Heck. 1995. (WHO/HRH/95.7. Unpublished). https://apps.who.int/iris/handle/10665/59441
18. Kaufman A, Scott MA, Andazola J, Fitzsimmons-Pattison D, Parajón L. Social accountability and graduate medical education. Fam Med. 2021;53(7):632–7. https://doi.org/10.22454/FamMed.2021.160888.

19. Barber C, van der Vleuten C, Leppink J, Chahine S. Social accountability frameworks and their implications for medical education and program evaluation: a narrative review. Acad Med. 2020;95(12):1945–54. https://doi.org/10.1097/ACM.0000000000003731.
20. Boelen C, Woollard R. Social accountability: the extra leap to excellence for educational institutions. Med Teach. 2011;33(8):614–9. https://doi.org/10.3109/0142159X.2011.590248.
21. Fung OW, Ying Y. Twelve tips to center social accountability in undergraduate medical education. Med Teach. 2021;22:1–7. https://doi.org/10.1080/0142159X.2021.1948983.
22. Muirhead L, Brasher S, Broadnax D, Chandler R. A framework for evaluating SDOH curriculum integration. J Prof Nurs. 2022;39:1–9. https://doi.org/10.1016/j.profnurs.2021.12.004.
23. Frye AW, Hemmer PA. Program evaluation models and related theories: AMEE Guide No. 67. Med Teach. 2012;34(5):e288–99. https://doi.org/10.3109/0142159X.2012.668637.
24. Kirkpatrick D. Great ideas revisited. Train Dev. 1996;50(1):54.
25. Nouraey P, Al-Badi A, Riasati MJ, Maata RL. Educational program and curriculum evaluation models: a mini systematic review of the recent trends. UJER. 2020;8(9):4048–55. https://doi.org/10.13189/ujer.2020.080930.
26. Proctor E, Silmere H, Raghavan R, et al. Outcomes for implementation research: conceptual distinctions, measurement challenges, and research agenda. Admin Pol Ment Health. 2011;38(2):65–76. https://doi.org/10.1007/s10488-010-0319-7.
27. Glasgow RE, Vogt TM, Boles SM. Evaluating the public health impact of health promotion interventions: the RE-AIM framework. Am J Public Health. 1999;89(9):1322–7. https://doi.org/10.2105/AJPH.89.9.1322.
28. Stufflebeam DL. The CIPP model for evaluation. Dordrecht: Kluwer Academic Publishers; 2003.
29. Stufflebeam DL, Shinkfield AJ. Systematic evaluation: a self-instructional guide to theory and practice, vol. 8. Cham: Springer Science & Business Media.
30. Buker M, Niklason G. Curriculum evaluation & improvement model. Published online; 2019. p. 19.
31. Phillips JJ. Return on investment in training and performance improvement programs. New York: Routledge; 2012.
32. McNamara C. Field guide to nonprofit program design, marketing and evaluation. Minneapolis: Authenticity Consulting; 2006.
33. Chen HT. A comprehensive typology for program evaluation. J Eval Clin Pract. 2016;17(2):121–30.

Aligning SDOH Pillars to Learning Outcomes and Assessments

7

Wanjira Kinuthia, Autherine Abiri, Jill B. Hamilton, and Adarsh Char

Learning Objectives

- Explain the relationship between learning outcomes and assessments within nursing courses.
- Use curriculum mapping strategies to identify constructively aligned SDOH content within individual nursing courses and curricula.
- Identify strategies for integrating assessments in SDOH pillars in nursing education.
- Apply constructive alignment principles to course design in nursing education.

Introduction

As the health system moves toward value-based models, the healthcare industry increasingly regards the social determinants of health (SDOH) as critical components in patient care. By focusing on the key features of well-being concerning healthcare, providers are taking a holistic view of patients and overall population health to enhance patient care, promote excellent outcomes, and drive value in healthcare provision [1].

The World Health Organization [2] defines the social determinants of health as "the non-medical factors that influence health outcomes. They are the conditions in which people are born, grow, work, live, and age, and the wider set of forces and

W. Kinuthia (✉) · A. Abiri · J. B. Hamilton
Nell Hodgson Woodruff School of Nursing, Emory University, Atlanta, GA, USA
e-mail: wkinuth@emory.edu; Autherine.abiri@emoryhealthcare.org; jbhamil@emory.edu

A. Char
Nell Hodgson Woodruff School of Nursing, Emory University, Atlanta, GA, USA

Full Tilt Ahead, Arlington, VA, USA
e-mail: achar2@emory.edu

systems shaping the conditions of daily life. These forces and systems include economic and development agendas, social norms, social policies, and political systems" [2]. WHO further indicates that social determinants of health influence health inequities. In countries with varying income levels, socioeconomic position affects their populations' quality of life and health. Research indicates that SDOH accounts for 30–55% of health outcomes [2], underscoring that SDOH is essential for improving health outcomes.

Integrating SDOH Pillars into the Nursing Curriculum

The current levels of health inequity cannot be relieved by just one healthcare profession alone. However, the nursing profession holds the capacity to address this significant challenge of the twenty-first century. According to Thornton and Persaud [3], nearly three million nurses are currently employed in the United States. Hence, the role of nurses in addressing health equity and the social determinants of health must be strengthened. Historically, SDOH pillars have not been purposefully integrated throughout most nursing education curricula. This has prevented graduating nurses from acquiring the knowledge necessary to assess and address these fundamental drivers of health.

Nursing programs can respond to the challenge of preparing nurses for social and health disparities, a call that has been met with support among professional nursing bodies.

Nurse educators can also contribute to fostering reflective practice and an understanding of the inequalities in healthcare [4]. In programs where the pillars are integrated, it is often done into the didactic components of a course. This approach is not necessarily effective in influencing future engagement and advocacy among the graduates [3, 5].

Opportunities for curricular integration should focus on educating nurses to identify the connections between SDOH and the challenges of their patients. Thus, connecting didactic material with meaningful clinical experiences in various settings is recommended. Kucherepa and O'Connell [5] suggest that working toward achieving cultural competence is a "dynamic, ongoing, developmental process that is a long-term commitment. Increasing one's cultural humility—the knowledge, skills, and applications—may improve patients' healthcare outcomes and satisfaction, simultaneously decreasing health disparities" in the SDOH pillars.

At Emory University's Nell Hodgson Woodruff School of Nursing (SON), the Four Pillars of SDOH are organized into four general areas: Social, Environmental, Cultural, and Political, as shown in Table 7.1. The School of Nursing's SDOH framework is unique in that, while other frameworks exist, nursing requires an approach that is "more pragmatic and comprehensive" to guide the way the social determinants are approached among the diverse populations the school serves. The framework must be helpful regardless of the setting or population [7]. At the SON, the faculty receive training on SDOH course integration and then rolls out the SDOH pillars. The process is implemented in the phases described in Chap. 5 on curriculum mapping.

Table 7.1 Based on the Emory Nursing's SDOH Framework course

Pillar	Definition and examples
Social conditions	Those conditions occur in society due to systemic racism, economic disparities, education gaps, and/or occupations that influence wellness Considerations: Access to education, financial resources, job opportunities, social support, language and health literacy, access to healthcare (use of preventive health services, primary care), and incarceration
Environmental	Physical environments have an outsized impact on individual and population health. The Emory Nursing SDOH Framework considers the following – Natural environment: Green space, buildings, bike lanes, sidewalks, lighting, trees, benches, exposure to toxic substances, access to foods that support healthy eating patterns – Natural resources: Climate, weather, air pollution, Naturally occurring social interactions/social connections, familial relationships, and social capital
Cultural	Customary beliefs, social norms, attitudes, values, and practices shared by a group of people (community or society) in a place and time can affect health outcomes Cultural conditions influencing SDOH include societal values, religion/spirituality, nursing values, interpersonal racism/discrimination, customs/behaviors, and identity (ethnicity, gender, sexual orientation)
Policy/law	The guidelines, principles, legislation, and activities affecting the living conditions conducive to the welfare of individuals', communities', and societies' quality of life This pillar considers the policies that affect social issues such as affordable/universal health insurance, child protection, abortion, guns, sex workers, LGBTQ issues (including same-sex marriage), Education/housing policies, recreational drugs, APRN restrictions (e.g., restriction on prescriptions, radiology, dispensing, and collaborating physician)

*Based on the Emory School of Nursing Course [6]

Constructive Alignment of SDOH

Changing healthcare needs requires different skill development approaches. This transformation dictates how nursing education evolves to meet these needs, and in these situations, constructive alignment can be advantageous [8]. Nursing is an applied academic and practice-based profession dependent on skill proficiency which requires skills and knowledge development in the cognitive, psychomotor, and affective domains. Nursing skills are taught using different strategies, for example, simulations in nursing skill development and problem-based learning. Additionally, skill development in nursing programs requires educators and clinicians to be involved in teaching the necessary skills through didactic and clinical learning experiences.

Biggs [9] defines constructive alignment as a teaching design that purposely plans what is intended for students to learn and how they should express this information in their learning. This information is outlined before teaching is initiated, and instruction is then designed to engage students in learning activities that optimize their chances of attaining those learning outcomes. Next, assessment tasks are designed to judge how well those outcomes have been attained. The work of Biggs is based on Tyler [10], who emphasized four critical areas: (1) What is the purpose

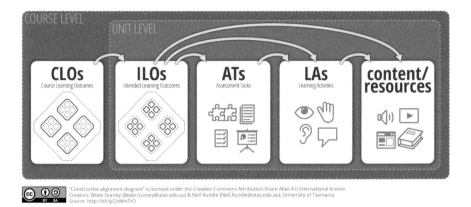

Fig. 7.1 A visual representation of Biggs [9] constructive alignment model. *University of Tasmania

that education seeks to attain? (2) How can educational experiences be provided to attain these purposes? (3) How these educational experiences should be effectively organized? and (4) How we can determine whether these purposes are attained [9, p. 6].

Figure 7.1, retrieved from the University of Tasmania website, visually represents constructive alignment based on Biggs [9] constructive alignment model. It denotes the relationship between Course Learning Outcomes (CLOs), unit-level Intended Learning Outcomes (ILOs), Assessment Tasks (ATs), Learning Activities (LAs), and learning content and resources [11].

Constructive alignment is regarded as a critical idea in higher education and is used in many courses [12, 13], where the entire planning system should be aligned with high cognitive level goals, as reflected in Bloom's Taxonomy [14–16]. Bloom's Taxonomy aims to help write learning goals and objectives that address what a student should be able to do upon completing an instructional unit. Using the appropriate action verb in the learning outcomes clarifies the order of thinking the student is expected to obtain [9, 12, 16].

There are six levels of cognitive learning based on the revised Bloom's Taxonomy [14, 16], and each level produces different outputs. These levels are *remembering, understanding, applying, analyzing, evaluating, and creating.* The levels are ordered from simple to complex and abstract to concrete as a progressive climb to higher-order thinking. These levels help develop learning outcomes because specific verbs fit best at each level. However, some action verbs are helpful at multiple levels, and specific learning outcomes and output are better associated with each taxonomy level.

Alignment in a course occurs when the learning activities help the students develop the knowledge and skills intended and measured by the assessment task [12]. A constructively aligned course links the effect of assessment to students' learning experiences rather than the assessment driving students [13, 17]. The basis of constructive alignment is that learning should be worthwhile and that assessment must enhance practical knowledge. That is, we know what we teach and how to improve it with assessment tasks [18, 19].

Constructive alignment is approached in the following order: (1) Identify the intended learning outcomes, which an action verb should guide; (2) Design assessment tasks to measure whether the learning outcomes have been attained; (3) Plan learning activities that enable students to develop the skills, knowledge, and understanding in the learning outcomes and measured by assessment; and (4) Select the content, such as topics, resource, and materials, examples that will support the learning activities. The verb in the learning outcomes becomes the link that aligns the learning outcome, teaching/learning activities, and assessment tasks [9, 20].

Formative assessments, also described as *assessments for learning*, are more diagnostic than evaluative. They monitor learning, provide ongoing feedback, and allow educators to adjust teaching methods and improve students' learning. Formative assessments test students' comprehension and understanding of knowledge or skills during teaching and learning to elicit feedback to support learning outcomes [21]. Generally, formative assessment strategies are quick to use and fit seamlessly into the lesson. The information is rarely graded, but descriptive feedback may accompany the assessment to notify the students if they have mastered a learning outcome or whether more practice is required. Examples of formative assessment are impromptu quizzes, anonymous polling, 1-min papers, peer assessments, concept maps, and research proposals or paper outlines for early feedback [22].

Summative assessments, also referred to as *assessments of learning*, are typically administered at the end of an instructional period, for example, the end of a project, module, course, semester, program, or academic year [23]. The assessments are used to evaluate student learning, acquisition of skills acquisition, and academic achievement and are generally defined by three criteria: (1) to determine whether and to what degree the students have learned the content they have been taught; (2) because they are given at the end of a specific period, they are evaluative, rather than diagnostic; and (3) they are recorded as scores that are factored into a student's academic record. Therefore, they provide a benchmark for checking students' progress, programs, and institutions. Examples of summative assessments in nursing programs include midterm and final exams, final papers, end-of-unit or chapter tests, and cumulative work such as final projects and portfolios [22].

Curriculum Mapping in Nursing Education

Ng [24] defines a curriculum as a roadmap or plan for learning. It includes what, why, how, when, and who concerning the design and delivery of a program and module. The curriculum consists of information on how modules are structured within a program and the alignment of each course relating to the course learning outcomes, teaching and learning strategies, and assessments. Curriculum mapping is a tool for organizing, managing, and evaluating curricula, using visual approaches, databases, or spreadsheets to manage and cross-reference course and program data

[25, 26]. The mapping process is often a response to expanding or refining professional standards and increasing pressures for course and accreditation [13].

Harden [27] and Plaza et al. [28] indicate that the primary function of curriculum maps in health-related programs is to make the curriculum more transparent and to illustrate the links between the components of the curriculum. The mapping exercise provides a broad overview of the curriculum and its intended learning outcomes to the various stakeholders. It requires a systematic analysis of the content of the courses in a curriculum [25]. Ideally, the curriculum map should include the critical components of a curriculum, such as, what is taught, when it is taught, how it is taught, and how it is assessed, and also demonstrate the relationships and nature of the connections between the key components. However, few published accounts of curriculum mapping projects in higher education [25, 26]. Curriculum maps in health-related programs are used to identify deficiencies in the curriculum, support the planning of assessment activities, and develop models to guide the assessment process [28].

In nursing education, developing the program curricula requires understanding the fundamentals of relevant curriculum design and competency-based [29]. Curriculum mapping in nursing is an evidence-based approach to curriculum design that promotes faculty collaboration and quality assurance in nursing education. Neville-Norton and Cantwell also reference the Institute of Medicine's call for transformation in nursing education which has witnessed a shift in nursing education and practice. The reform has also highlighted the need for nursing programs to develop and deliver curricula that promotes high skill and competency attainment for graduates. Further, as noted by Levin and Suhayda [30], nursing education is transitioning from a culture of individual faculty course design and facilitation to collegiality and collaboration. This collaboration is reflected in curriculum development that engages faculty in nursing programs in the curriculum design, instruction, and student learning assessment [31].

As noted by Porter [32], curriculum maps serve three primary purposes, which are to (1) identify whether the intended instructional content is being taught and what students learn; (2) demonstrate the links between critical components of the curriculum, which are learning outcomes, content, and assessment; and (3) examine various sections of the curriculum including learning resources, scheduling, and delivery modes. Porter [32] and Harden [27] describe a process for measuring the alignment between instruction content using three tools for measuring content and alignment: (1) instructor surveys; (2) content analyses of instructional resources like textbooks and syllabi; and (3) alignment indices that indicate the degree of overlap between standards, content, and assessment.

In nursing programs, curriculum mapping is viewed as a quality assurance process where program planners can visually demonstrate the teaching and learning process from beginning to end [29]. Additionally, curriculum mapping is viewed as a high-level tool for visualizing the alignment of program and course curricula to accreditation standards and national guidelines [29, 33]. The nursing program's professional standards for curriculum development are derived from major nursing organizations, including the American Nursing Association, American Association of Nurse Practitioners, and American Nurses Credentialing Center. Curriculum mapping is utilized for multiple purposes. This includes assessing existing nursing curricula for course alignment and gaps, developing new curricula, and revising nursing curricula [29, 30, 34].

Assessment in Nursing Education

In nursing education and practice, assessment is critical to obtaining information about student learning and evaluating their competencies and clinical performance. Assessment is also fundamental to monitoring and evaluating the quality of instructional and healthcare programs. Program effectiveness can be measured by evaluating outcomes achieved by nursing students, graduates, and patients and decisions about areas needing improvement [35, p. 3].

Ensuring accountability for the quality of education and information for program evaluation and accreditation is integral to program assessment [29]. Assessments should provide important valid, and reliable data for determining learning outcomes. Although nurse programs routinely assess students' progress in learning outcomes and developing clinical competencies, measuring students' achievement in a course is essential. Effective assessment strategies should therefore provide the data to instructors to determine if students have achieved the outcomes and developed the necessary clinical competencies.

Nursing programs use various assessment strategies, including tests, papers, written assignments, projects, case studies, small-group activities, simulation-based assessments, oral presentations, ePortfolios, observations of performance, and objective structured clinical examinations [35]. Many nursing programs also use commercial tests as the students' progress through the curriculum. These tests aim to identify gaps in students' learning and prepare them to take the National Council Licensure Examinations, the NCLEX-RN®, and NCLEX-PN® [35].

Reviewing Nursing Courses for Alignment

Before integrating the SDOH pillars into their courses, faculty were guided on SDOH and teaching strategies for their consideration. This was done through an online asynchronous training course. A curriculum map that aimed to identify whether there was constructive alignment between learning outcomes, assessments, and activities was developed and conducted with MSN and MN courses in 2021. Once the baseline map was completed, as described in Chap. 5, the mapping team began the process of individual course analysis. We reviewed 16 courses in the MSN program and nine courses in the Post-Licensure program, or what used to be known as the MSN program. Learning outcomes, assessments, and activities were reviewed for alignment within Canvas, the SON's online Learning Management System (LMS). Course review encompassed didactic courses and excluded labs, clinical, and practicum courses.

Table 7.2 Course review matrix

Course title					
Assessment (title)	Type	Level	SDOH pillar	Assignment information/SDOH content covered	Notes
For example, quiz 1	For example, discussion forum	For example, advanced	For example, social and cultural	Brief description of the assignment	
For example, professional nursing paper	For example, case study	For example, intermediate	For example, law/policy	Brief description of the assignment	

These questions guided individual course reviews and analyses:

1. To what extent are assignments specific to SDOH integrated into the courses?
2. When are assignments integrated into the courses, and at what level on Bloom's Taxonomy are they assessed?

We reviewed each course using a two-phase approach. The first phase used a qualitative approach to holistically examine the course syllabi and module contents to determine whether and how SDOH pillars were included in each course. The analysis also examined whether the course and module learning outcomes aligned with assignments. The metrics we looked at included course artifacts such as textbook chapters, articles, PowerPoint slides, quizzes, exams, assignments, recorded video lectures, case studies, empirical articles, papers, policy papers, discussion forums, policy briefs, and external links to resources, and instructional videos. The artifacts varied based on individual course goals and design.

The second phase, which was quantitative, documented the number of assignments that specifically integrated SDOH pillars. The in-depth analysis of the assignments was done using a course mapping matrix. The levels of the assignments were categorized based on Bloom's Taxonomy, i.e., beginning (remembering and understanding), intermediate (applying and analyzing), and advanced (evaluating and creating) [15, 16]. As shown in Table 7.2, the in-depth assignment review also identified which pillars were embedded in the assignments. Using the matrix as a template and guide coincided with the aforementioned qualitative approach. The mapping committee worked with faculty members and instructional designers to comprehensively carry out the curriculum mapping and examination of alignment of the learning outcomes with assessment.

Findings in the Nursing Courses Analyses

All courses in the SON include the specific SON SDOH objective in the syllabus at the course level. However, not all courses had SDOH learning outcomes at the module level. The SON SDOH objectives read as follows:

Pre-Licensure: Students will define and/or assess the influences of SDOH (cultural, social, environmental, and political) on illness and wellness in healthcare at the individual, family, community, and societal levels.

Post-licensure: Students will evaluate and apply evidence-based knowledge about the influences of SDOH (cultural, social, environmental, and political) on illness and wellness related to advanced practice and research with diverse populations at the individual, family, community, and societal levels.

Courses that included SDOH learning outcomes mainly did so at the intermediate (applying and analyzing) and advanced (evaluating and creating) level [15, 16]. Examples of learning outcomes at the course level in one course were: (1) Describe factors that influence the healthcare outcomes and environments of individuals and families, including culture, spirituality, genetics, environment, and information technology; (2) Use the principles of illness prevention and health promotion in planning care; and (3) Engage in ethical reasoning and identify strategies to promote advocacy, collaboration, and social justice for application to simulated learning experiences and the clinical setting. Examples of learning outcomes at the module level in another course were: (1) Discuss the ethical and legal implications of nursing as a profession and discipline; (2) Recognize policy advocacy and activism as a moral duty of nurses and nursing; and (3) Frame the moral story of policy issues through the lens of nursing. In these courses, the learning outcomes were mainly aligned with the assessments.

The levels of assignments were categorized as either beginning, intermediate, or advanced. The categorization was based on Bloom's Taxonomy of what the students should be able to do by the end of the course. Courses that included SDOH assignment outcomes did so mainly at the intermediate or advanced levels. The assignments were created at the beginning level in a few courses, particularly in quizzes. Most courses included at least one assignment related to the SDOH pillars; in most courses, there were at least two to four.

The SDOH pillars covered in each course vary based on the course goals and content, but the social and cultural pillars were the most recurrent in the courses. There were also overlaps with the social and policy, with the environmental pillar being the least captured. Formative and summative assessments covering social pillars assessed students on topics such as access to primary healthcare based on race and age, financial and economic disparities, and health literacy. Table 7.3 is an example of one course that we reviewed. In another course, the topics covered significant historical issues impacting healthcare. The assignments required the students to explain how this occurrence relates to current healthcare disparities and the implications for how race has developed as a category in healthcare. Next, the students had to apply this information to their future roles as Advanced Practice Registered Nurses (APRNs). In yet another course, assignments on cultural pillars included topics and assignments on religion, spirituality, nursing, societal values, and interpersonal discrimination based on ethnicity, gender, and sexual orientation. As an additional example, another course was designed to have assignments based

Table 7.3 Example of a reviewed course

Course title					
Assessment (title)	Type	Level	SDOH pillar	Assignment information/SDOH content covered	Notes
Breaking difficult news video	Video recording	Advanced	Social; cultural	Students will record and upload themselves presenting "difficult news" along with a self-evaluation	
Annotated bibliography	Writing assignment	Advanced	Policy/law; social; cultural	Students select a list of articles to review from a resource and prepare an annotated bibliography. Topic examples are Health systems & policy; improving care for seriously ill hospitalized patients; Provision of spiritual support to patients with advanced cancer; Cost saving, and Medicare	
Final exam	Quiz	Advanced	Policy/law; social; cultural	Questions include Landmark bioethics legal cases, aging, and culture	

on understanding LGBTQIA+ concepts and disparities, communicating effectively with LGBTQIA+ patients, and addressing sexual orientation, gender identity, and health disparities through clinical care.

Law/policy topics and assignments in several post-licensure courses included coverage on social security, health insurance, assisted death, Affordable Care Act, Medicare, financial and economic implications of healthcare, regulations for running a healthcare business, medical billing and coding guidelines, child and elder protection, affordable housing, quality education, sex work, abortion, and guns. Students had to use their nursing expertise to communicate their support or opposition to identified issues through elected officials or position papers.

Courses that relied on active recall or those that covered quantitative content tended to have lower coverage of SDOH pillar assignments than those that addressed survey topics. For example, Pharmacology for Nursing Practice and Physiology/Pathophysiology for Nursing Practice covered fewer SDOH pillars than the Art and Science of Nursing Practice course or post-licensure courses like Leadership and Professional Nursing Is Nursing Issues and Trends. Although the environmental pillar was the least embedded, topics included access to foods that support healthy eating patterns, green spaces, exposure to toxic substances, air pollution, and climate.

Many assignments covered multiple pillars. For example, a policy brief assignment required students to synthesize topics related to social, cultural, and policy pillars. For instance, in one assignment, students were asked to write an informed policy brief compiled throughout the semester to address and provide a nursing recommendation or solution and rationale for their selected topic related to a political, economic, sociocultural, and/or technological context. Although many courses covered SDOH pillars, the content was not necessarily included in the assignments.

In a majority of the courses, assignments were primarily designed in the form of discussion forum questions, case study analyses, video analyses, essays, external course activities, group assignments, oral presentations, writing assignments (papers), exams, quizzes, surveys, video recordings, video analyses, debates, policy briefs, op-eds, blogs, speeches, social media posts, worksheets, and synthesis matrices. The most common forms were discussion questions, writing assignments, case studies, and quizzes.

Summary

The course review process allowed us to answer the two guiding questions regarding the extent to which assignments specifically integrated SDOH pillars and at what level the level on Bloom's Taxonomy was assessed. That is, how aligned the learning objectives were to the course assignments, both formative and summative. We found that learning activities courses often rely on discussions and case studies centered on SDOH topics. Overlaps in social, cultural, and policy pillars often occur. Hence, assignments also incorporate the themes into the assignments.

Because the environmental pillar was the least addressed, it would be beneficial to seek ways to integrate it, for example, by combining pertinent topics and examples alongside social and law/policy pillars. Identifying and revising courses where SDOH pillars are addressed to a lesser extent in the assignments would help students see the connection between the learning outcomes, course content, and assignments. Highlighting the linkages also establishes whether the learning outcomes are being met and also helps to motivate students to see how the information will be of value to them as healthcare providers.

As seen in this chapter, there is often significant variability and completeness in the coverage of the issues in the SDOH pillars. Including more experiential and didactic and experiential learning experiences to develop competencies and identify and resolve SDOH curriculum gaps is essential. It is also considered an effective teaching methodology for increasing awareness of the determinants by linking learning outcomes to the assessments. Integrating the social determinants into the courses has been valuable in helping faculty members at the SON innovatively integrate the pillars in the specific courses they teach. The approach also helps to demonstrate to the students that the SDOH pillars are not isolated from the care they provide to their patients. Along with daily reflective practice, understanding inequalities as a challenge that concerns the healthcare profession can also advance nurses as critical transformative care providers. By doing so, we can better address the inequities in the healthcare system.

Reflection

– The curriculum mapping process can be instrumental in also determining whether a course is constructively aligned, and the process can be carried out simultaneously.
– Course alignment is best addressed during course planning and continuously improved with subsequent course offerings.
– Integrating learning objectives, assessments, and SDOH content within each course gradually requires ongoing sustainability revisions.
– Engaging key stakeholders, including faculty, leadership, and students, is necessary for receiving and implementing feedback in periodic curriculum reviews.

Chapter Review Questions

1. What are the components of constructive alignment?
   (a) Learning outcomes
   (b) Teaching and learning activities
   (c) Assessments
   (d) *All the above*
2. Identify the correct order of the six levels of cognitive learning based on the revised Bloom's Taxonomy from the lowest to highest order.
   (a) *Remembering, understanding, applying, analyzing, evaluating, and creating.*
   (b) Understanding, remembering, applying, analyzing, creating, evaluating
   (c) Creating, evaluating, remembering, understanding, applying, analyzing
   (d) Understanding, remembering, applying, analyzing, creating, evaluating
   (e) Remembering, creating, evaluating, understanding, applying, analyzing
3. In which order is constructive alignment approached?
   (a) (i) Design assessment tasks; (ii) identify the intended learning outcomes; (iii) Plan learning activities; (iv) Select the content
   (b) *(i) Identify the intended learning outcomes; (ii) Design assessment tasks; (iii) Plan learning activities (iv); elect the content*
   (c) (i) Identify the intended learning outcomes; (ii) Design assessment tasks; (iii) Plan learning activities; and (iv) Select the content
   (d) (i) Select the content; identify the intended learning outcomes; (ii; iii) Plan learning activities; (iv) Design assessment tasks
4. WHO research indicates that SDOH accounts between _____ of health outcomes underscoring that SDOH is essential for improving health outcomes.
   (a) 10 and 15%
   (b) 80 and 85%
   (c) *30 and 55%*
   (d) 50 and 75%
5. According to the findings, courses that rely on active recall tended to have lower coverage of SDOH pillar assignments than those that address survey topics.
   (a) *True*
   (b) False

Answers
- 1. (d), 2. (a), 3. (b), 4. (c), 5. (a)

References

1. Catalyst N. Social determinants of health (SDOH). NEJM Catal. 2017;3(6). https://catalyst.nejm.org/doi/full/10.1056/cat.17.0312.
2. WHO. Social determinants of health. World Health Organization; 2008. Retrieved 25 May from https://www.who.int/health-topics/social-determinants-of-health#tab=tab_1
3. Thornton M, Persaud S. Preparing today's nurses: social determinants of health and nursing education. Online J Issues Nurs. 2018;23(3). https://ojin.nursingworld.org/MainMenuCategories/ANAMarketplace/ANAPeriodicals/OJIN/TableofContents/Vol-23-2018/No3-Sept-2018/Social-Determinants-of-Health-Nursing-Education.html.
4. Rozendo CA, Salas AS, Cameron B. A critical review of social and health inequalities in the nursing curriculum. Nurse Educ Today. 2017;50:62–71.
5. Kucherepa U, O'Connell MB. Self-assessment of cultural competence and social determinants of health within a first-year required pharmacy course. Pharmacy. 2021;10(1):6. https://doi.org/10.3390/pharmacy10010006.
6. Emory. Emory School of Nursing's SDOH framework. Emory School of Nursing. 2020. Retrieved 25 May from https://rise.articulate.com/share/ED2wyDMDBhUy53UxcbIoi50FC9Y8EUdF#/lessons/GQxbm6QPXkN-1Lsjh_bPjjHiluPgtq7y
7. Auchmutey P. Determinant determination. Emory Nursing Magazine, Autumn. 2021. https://emorynursingmagazine.emory.edu/issues/2021/autumn/features/determinant-determination/index.html
8. Joseph S, Juwah C. Using constructive alignment theory to develop nursing skills curricula. Nurse Educ Pract. 2012;12(1):52–9.
9. Biggs J. Constructive alignment in university teaching. HERDSA Rev High Educ. 2014;1:5–22.
10. Tyler RW. Basic principles of curriculum and instruction. Chicago: University of Chicago Press; 1946.
11. University of Tasmania. Teaching and learning: constructive alignment. University of Tasmania; n.d. Retrieved 26 May from https://www.teaching-learning.utas.edu.au/unit-design/constructive-alignment
12. Kandlbinder P, Peseta T. Key concepts in postgraduate certificates in higher education teaching and learning in Australasia and the United Kingdom. Int J Acad Dev. 2009;14(1):19–31.
13. Kertesz J. U-map: beyond curriculum mapping. Adv Scholarsh Teach Learn. 2015;2(1):16–34.
14. Anderson LW, Krathwohl DR, (eds). A taxonomy for learning, teaching, and assessing: a revision of Bloom's taxonomy of educational objectives. 2004.
15. Bloom BS. Taxonomy of educational objectives: the classification of educational goals. Cognitive domain. 1956.
16. Krathwohl DR. A revision of Bloom's taxonomy: an overview. Theory Pract. 2002;41(4):212–8.
17. Biggs J. Enhancing teaching through constructive alignment. High Educ. 1996;32(3):347–64.
18. Bell C, Simmons A, Martin E, McKenzie C, McLeod J, McCoombe S. Competent with patients and populations: integrating public health into a medical program. BMC Med Educ. 2019;19(1):1–9.
19. Boud D. Assessment and learning–unlearning bad habits of assessment. Conference on effective assessment at University, University of Queensland. 1998.
20. Biggs J. What the student does: teaching for enhanced learning. High Educ Res Dev. 1999;18(1):57–75.
21. Ali L. The design of curriculum, assessment and evaluation in higher education with constructive alignment. J Educ e-Learn Res. 2018;5(1):72–8.

22. Dixson DD, Worrell FC. Formative and summative assessment in the classroom. Theory Pract. 2016;55(2):153–9.
23. Allal L. Assessment and the regulation of learning. In: International encyclopedia of education, vol. 3; 2010. p. 348–52.
24. Ng V. Re-designing the architecture curriculum through the lens of graduate capabilities. In: Preparing 21st century teachers for teach less, learn more (TLLM) pedagogies. IGI Global; 2020. p. 221–42.
25. Archambault SG, Masunaga J. Curriculum mapping as a strategic planning tool. J Libr Adm. 2015;55(6):503–19.
26. Bell CE, Ellaway RH, Rhind SM. Getting started with curriculum mapping in a veterinary degree program. J Vet Med Educ. 2009;36(1):100–6.
27. Harden R. Curriculum mapping: a tool for transparent and authentic teaching and learning. AMEE Guide No. 21. Med Teach. 2001;23(2):123–37.
28. Plaza CM, Draugalis JR, Slack MK, Skrepnek GH, Sauer KA. Curriculum mapping in program assessment and evaluation. Am J Pharm Educ. 2007;71(2):20.
29. Neville-Norton M, Cantwell S. Curriculum mapping in nursing education: a case study for collaborative curriculum design and program quality assurance. Teach Learn Nurs. 2019;14(2):88–93.
30. Levin PF, Suhayda R. Transitioning to the DNP: ensuring integrity of the curriculum through curriculum mapping. Nurse Educ. 2018;43(3):112–4.
31. Hermann CP, Head BA, Black K, Singleton K. Preparing nursing students for interprofessional practice: the interdisciplinary curriculum for oncology palliative care education. J Prof Nurs. 2016;32(1):62–71.
32. Porter AC. Measuring the content of instruction: uses in research and practice. Educ Res. 2002;31(7):3–14.
33. Arafeh S. Curriculum mapping in higher education: a case study and proposed content scope and sequence mapping tool. J Furth High Educ. 2016;40(5):585–611.
34. Beckham R, Riedford K, Hall M. Course mapping: expectations visualized. J Nurse Pract. 2017;13(10):e471–6.
35. Oermann MH, Gaberson KB. Evaluation and testing in nursing education. In: Evaluation and testing in nursing education. Springer Publishing Company; 2016. p. 3–22. https://doi.org/10.1891/9780826135759.0001

Lessons Learned

8

Jill B. Hamilton, Adarsh Char, Linda McCauley,
Autherine Abiri, Laura Kimble, Lalita Kaligotla,
Beth Ann Swan, and Kristy Martyn

Learning Objectives

1. Describe areas of success with integration of SDOH content into the curriculum.
2. Describe the challenges of integration of SDOH content into curriculum.
3. List 2–3 recommendations for faculty success with integration of SDOH into curriculum.

Introduction

Our school-wide initiative to fully integrate SDOH concepts throughout all didactic and clinical courses began in August 2019. At the time of this writing, the process outlined in this text has taken 3 years and we are still working toward steps to evaluate, revise, and refine this initiative. We detail in the "Lessons Learned" chapter the challenges encountered and successes over the past 3 years and our plans for revision and refinement of this school-wide initiative to fully integrate SDOH concepts into our nursing curriculum.

J. B. Hamilton (✉) · L. McCauley · A. Abiri · L. Kimble · L. Kaligotla · B. A. Swan ·
K. Martyn
Nell Hodgson Woodruff School of Nursing, Emory University, Atlanta, GA, USA
e-mail: jbhamil@emory.edu; Linda.mccauley@emory.edu; Autherine.abiri@emoryhealth-care.org; Laura.porter.kimble@emory.edu; Lalita.kaligotla@emory.edu; Beth.ann.swan@emory.edu; Kristy.k.martyn@emory.edu

A. Char
Nell Hodgson Woodruff School of Nursing, Emory University, Atlanta, GA, USA

Full Tilt Ahead, Arlington, VA, USA
e-mail: achar2@emory.edu

As with any major school-wide initiative, we attribute our success to date to the following strategies presented in this chapter:

- *Leadership and administrative support from the highest level of administration who realized the importance of SDOH to the education of all of our nursing students.*
- *Faculty development and training through online courses and faculty workshops.*
- *Curriculum Committee engagement and support of the process.*
- *Nursing faculty awareness and value for SDOH in nursing education*

Administrative support from the dean for this SDOH curriculum initiative through:

1. Top-level support and consistent communication from the leadership team who consistently and clearly articulated the value of educating Emory School of Nursing students at all levels on SDOH as a necessity for the delivery of optimal care to the diverse populations and communities that we serve.
2. Ensuring that the School of Nursing Leadership Team was supportive with this initiative. The Dean assured regular and ongoing placement of SDOH on the agendas of All Faculty meetings, Curriculum Committee meetings, and the Dean's Educational Council meetings. Because SDOH was an important agenda item throughout the planning and execution of educational strategies to integrate SDOH throughout the curriculum, we were able to obtain critical, formative input, and feedback during all phases of SDOH integration.
3. Strategically appointing and placing key SDOH leaders in prominent roles on committees and leadership councils. These key leaders included the Associate Dean for Education, Chair of Curriculum Committee, Assistant Dean of Equity, Diversity, and Inclusion, and a Senior Faculty Fellow of SDOH and Health Disparities.
4. The Senior Faculty Fellow of SDOH and Health Disparities used allocated effort/release time to lead faculty development, coordinate implementation efforts of other faculty, and monitor efforts to evaluate faculty teaching of SDOH content.

Challenges to administrative support   In the early phases of this initiative, the multipronged work of faculty development, implementation and evaluation of teaching, and student outcomes was complex and time intensive. Initially, the Senior Fellow developed the SDOH framework that was adopted and shared with faculty at all levels as the SDOH foundation for the school. In order to facilitate integration of SDOH in the curriculum across all levels (doctoral, masters, and bachelor's programs) it was determined that we needed three SDOH core teams focused on: (1) Faculty Development, (2) Design and Implementation, and (3) Evaluation. A lead faculty was appointed for each core team. Progress was made in developing objectives for every course in the curriculum and piloting of integration with a group of prelicensure students. However, it became apparent that one leader was needed to oversee the three core areas to ensure integration of SDOH in the curriculum across levels and regular communication with school leadership and faculty.

A reset plan was established by the Dean and the Senior Faculty Fellow of SDOH. It was decided that the Senior Faculty Fellow of SDOH would lead of all three leadership cores with administrative support. Overseeing the three core areas involved regular and close monitoring of the process with a focus on expanding integration of SDOH across all education programs. An administrative staff was assigned to assist with scheduling meetings, recording meetings, and storing documents (presentations, SDOH literature) on our one drive system for easy access among faculty.

Recommendation for administrative supports

1. A designated SDOH lead person with the authority and effort for oversight of all phases of faculty development, implementation, and evaluation of SDOH content into curriculum. The lead person needs to have the seniority and experience to know the different faculty in the school and the different curricular components. We chose to have our designated SDOH lead person come from the faculty and not be a person holding an established administrative role.
2. Administrative staff personnel to support the SDOH lead person.
3. Regular team meetings that included the Dean who kept her leadership team informed.
4. Release time/effort allocated for a designated SDOH lead person.
5. Clear communication from Dean and SDOH Faculty Fellow to Program Directors and faculty that education to alleviate health disparities and deliver optimal care will require the integration of social determinants into our nursing curriculum at all levels.
6. Engagement of faculty, including ongoing communication via faculty and curriculum meetings.

Faculty Development with the assistance of a designated faculty team and Instructional Design Director. Major components of faculty development included:

1. A self-paced SDOH Canvas Course with CE credit, made accessible within our School's learning management system, Canvas. This course was developed in consultation with an Instructional Design expert (see Chap. 3). This course included a pre and posttest of SDOH content, and Discussion Group Assignment option section for faculty to share discussion posts with exemplars of ways in which SDOH was integrated into their courses through student assignments. These discussion posts were subsequently downloaded, placed into categories according to SDOH Pillar (Social, Cultural, Environmental, and Policy) with the final product being a Faculty Handbook for faculty to use as a resource as they integrated SDOH content into their courses.

2. Individual faculty consultations with the SDOH lead and Instructional Design Expert to answer questions on content for a specific course. These consultations were provided to faculty on a weekly schedule of open hours.
3. Faculty teaching/learning sessions to answer questions and making suggestions for student assignments according to SDOH Pillars.

Challenges to faculty development Challenges were found with faculty attendance in the SDOH Canvas Course, individual consultations, and teaching/learning sessions. Although the response from faculty to the SDOH Canvas Course was extremely positive with high engagement, not all faculty participated. Inadvertently, part-time clinical instructors were not included in emails announcing the availability of the course. Additionally, since the course was not mandated, not all faculty accessed the course. Secondly, the faculty did not respond well to the individual consultations to address SDOH into their courses and only a fraction of the faculty attended the teaching/learning session. These challenges were not unanticipated. Faculty frequently cite a lack of time to attend online professional courses or may believe that SDOH is not relevant to the courses they teach. Follow up with individual faculty was needed to ensure that all faculty teaching our students were aware of this school-wide initiative.

Recommendation for faculty development Optimally, faculty teaching courses across all levels of nursing students should be fully engaged in the integration of SDOH into the curriculum. Suggestions might include:

1. Engagement with faculty development activities should be a requirement. Perhaps attendance to faculty development activities could be linked to annual performance reviews and merit increases.
2. A requirement for engagement in SDOH faculty development educational offerings should be for faculty at all levels including part-time clinical faculty.
3. Monthly offerings of workshops and lunch and learn sessions with smaller groups of faculty of didactic and clinical courses and/or clusters of faculty around core content. This frequent offering would provide more flexibility for faculty attendance.
4. Offerings of workshops and lunch and learn sessions with smaller groups of part-time clinical faculty.
5. On demand access providing support and consultation with SDOH lead faculty through monthly open office hours.
6. Designating courses as including specific content on SDOH as being SDOH focused. Turning the incentive from something a faculty perceives they "have" to do to a courses designation that faculty values could be a powerful incentive.

Curriculum Committee Engaged and Supportive of the Process Very early in the process of integration of SDOH into the curriculum, the SDOH lead faculty, members of the Dean's Administrative team, met regularly with the Chair of the Curriculum Committee and Program Directors. During these meetings:

1. The Emory School of Nursing 4-Pillar SDOH framework and a draft of course objectives based on this framework for class syllabi were presented for discussion and feedback.
2. Using the existing Curriculum Committee structure, SDOH objectives for class syllabi were approved and the Chair of Curriculum Committee led the process of SDOH course objectives approved during an all-faculty meeting.
3. Curriculum Committee structure was necessary to ensure that the process was conducted according to the bylaws of the faculty governance structure in the School of Nursing.

Challenges to curriculum committee engagement Getting the support of a large group of Curriculum Committee members to agree on an SDOH framework and course objectives presented a challenge and were time intensive. However, this buy-in was a critical step to obtain all faculty support for adopting the Emory School of Nursing 4-Pillar SDOH framework and objectives as a guide for course content. We were successful with the Curriculum Committee's adoption of the framework and course objectives but the mapping of SDOH content into individual courses was extremely time intensive, requiring a different approach.

Recommendation to curriculum committee engagement

1. Obtain input and support from the Curriculum Committee Chair and key members and/or other faculty governance groups overseeing the curriculum in the very early phases of SDOH integration.
2. Assess the usual functioning of the committee and appropriately judge whether the existing committee structure has the time, resources, and expertise to successfully complete the required elements of SDOH content integration.
3. Mapping of courses for SDOH content may be too burdensome for the existing Curriculum Committee Structure and require an ad hoc team.
4. Appoint an ad hoc team with time and skill set to collaborate with program directors to map SDOH in individual courses necessary to avoid redundancy of SDOH content.

Nursing Faculty Awareness and Value for SDOH in Nursing Education Perhaps the greatest factor of success with the integration of SDOH into the curriculum was from faculty who either recognized and/or valued the incorporation of this content into their courses. We consider ourselves fortunate to have had a faculty that recognized the importance of SDOH content in the education of nursing students, Generally, faculty whom, although extremely busy and had planned out their syllabi for the semester, were willing to make the adjustments necessary to modify their courses to include SDOH content. Additionally, these faculty, with limited time and bandwidth, had already prepared their syllabus and outlined their course within our learning management system. Examples of the creativity of faculty with the integration of SDOH content into the curriculum are detailed in Chap. 5. Exemplars included:

1. Faculty exemplified a degree of creativity with the incorporation of Emory-wide resources from the Humanities (Arts and Social Justice Grants) that permitted faculty to launch new pedagogical initiatives that extended classroom learning to include community collaborations and ways in which these communities use the arts to express social justice issues.
2. Faculty demonstrated how SDOH content could be included in a content-dense course in our Pharmacology course. This faculty member who has taught traditional pharmacology content for many years incorporated content focused on racism as a SDOH factor that influenced best practices with the administration of medications among racial/ethnic populations. Specifically, faculty focused on the integration of SDOH conditions into courses focused on foundational knowledge of pharmacology as well as pharmacokinetics and pharmacodynamics across the lifespan. The NHWSN SDOH Four Pillar Framework was a guide to student learning the influences of SDOH within pharmacology and patient health.
3. Faculty demonstrated creativity in teaching with the development of a simulation scenario incorporating SDOH. The modification within an existing simulation course was informed by a compilation of student reflections during a community-based immersion with immigrant farmers in a small town in the Southern region of Georgia.

Challenges to faculty awareness and value of SDOH As with any organizational change, there were faculty who found it difficult to modify some clinical courses and course assignments to integrate SDOH content. The difficulty was related to the time required to modify courses to integrate this additional SDOH content. Initially, faculty expressed concern that they were being asked to add additional content and were uncertain of ways to modify courses without deleting content believed critical to their courses.

Recommendation to faculty awareness and value of SDOH Faculty development materials and learning sessions should include support and guidance to modify assignments so that faculty are not stressed with the addition or deletion of traditional content in order to integrate SDOH into courses. A broader issue is how to let go of traditional content that has served nursing well for decades, but still has left us with critical gaps in knowledge as the evidence grows of the significance of social, political, and cultural factors in achieving optimal health.

Summary

Our efforts to include integrate SDOH into our nursing curricula continue. While these efforts have been challenging and labor intensive, overall, the NHWSN community embraces the value of SDOH and is committed to sustaining this focus. As nursing education advances with new ideas and initiatives, such as the AACN Essentials and competency-based education, the School is committed to finding ways to keep our SDOH Framework, the 4 Pillars, and the ongoing integration and evaluation process at the forefront.